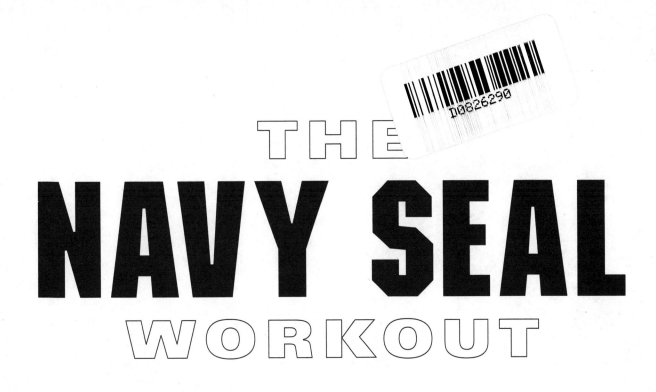

THE NAVY SEAL WORKOUT

THE NAVY SEAL WORKOUT

THE COMPLETE TOTAL-BODY FITNESS PROGRAM

MARK DE LISLE
U.S. NAVY SEAL

McGraw·Hill

New York   Chicago   San Francisco   Lisbon   London   Madrid   Mexico City
Milan   New Delhi   San Juan   Seoul   Singapore   Sydney   Toronto

The McGraw·Hill Companies

Library of Congress Cataloging-in-Publication Data

De Lisle, Mark.
    The Navy SEAL workout : the complete total-body fitness program / Mark De Lisle.
       p.   cm.
    ISBN 0-8092-2902-1
    1. Exercise.   2. Physical fitness.   3. United States.   4. Navy.
    5. SEALs.   I. Title.
    GV481.D395   1998
    613.7′1—dc21
                              97-38946
                              CIP

17 18 19 20 QVS/QVS 13

Printed in the United States of America

ISBN 0-8092-2902-1

Cover and interior photos by Birch Photography

McGraw-Hill books are available at special quantity discounts to use as premiums and sales promotions, or for use in corporate training programs. For more information, please write to the Director of Special Sales, Professional Publishing, McGraw-Hill, Two Penn Plaza, New York, NY 10121-2298. Or contact your local bookstore.

Consult a physician before you begin this or any strenuous exercise program or diet modification, especially if you have, or suspect that you may have, heart disease, high blood pressure, diabetes, or any other adverse medical conditions.

Warning: If you feel faint or dizzy at any time while performing any portion of this training program, stop immediately and seek medical evaluation.

The author and publisher disclaim any liability, personal or professional, resulting from the misapplication of any training procedure described in this publication.

Printed on acid-free paper.

"After having my baby, I didn't have time to go to the gym. I was afraid I'd never fit back into my old clothes. I ordered your book and was able to work out right at home. In less than four months I lost 5" in my waist and 3" in my hips. My old clothes fit better than before. I particularly benefited from the abdominal workout, which made me sore in muscles I had never felt before. I just want to thank you for providing me with a workout that I can use in the convenience of my own home."

—Sherie Anderson
Sacramento, California

"Your program is the best strength-training routine I have ever done. It would take me a year to gain with weights what I have achieved in six months with your program. The mental benefits are too long to list."

—Daniel O'Neil
Alberta, Canada

"I wanted to tell you how much I am enjoying your book—it is really fantastic! The program is phenomenal. It is a no-nonsense approach to fitness that anyone can use anywhere, anytime."

—Candace Cartwright
Leander, Texas

"I found your Navy SEAL training program to be outstanding. It is a complete exercise program that can be performed at home without paying for expensive gyms or heavy equipment. Those who apply themselves to your exercise program will obtain the best physical condition possible."

—Luis Pedro Aris
Brazil

"I have been following your Navy SEAL exercise program for over a year. It affords me greater conditioning and endurance than a conventional weight training schedule, without the debilitating effects. In addition, it has improved my coordination and dynamic strength considerably."

—Bruce MacTavish
Pasadena, California

"I'd like to take this opportunity to say 'thank you!' Your Navy SEAL training program has me in the best shape of my life. I began your program in June, after receiving a transfer to F.C.I. Cumberland, which has no weights—all I had worked out with for many years. I went from 185 lb. of bulk to 154 lb. of lean, cut, hard body. Many guys watch me work out and think it's easy until they try it. I'm proud to say I broke them down."

—*Leonard Giso*
Cumberland, Maryland

"*The Navy SEAL Workout* is the best purchase I think I've ever made. I went on a diet about a year ago and lost 40 lb., but no matter how much I worked out I just couldn't bulk up until I bought Mark De Lisle's book."

—*Grant Turnage*
Los Angeles, California

"Nobody said exercise has to be complicated. And nobody I know has designed a simpler, more practical training program than Mark De Lisle's."

—*Ken McAlpine*
Writer, *Outside* magazine

"I am a women's volleyball coach at the University of Wisconsin. I was a coach for the U.S. Men's National Team in the 1992 Olympics. Mark De Lisle has captured the magic of the Navy SEAL fitness program and presented it in a format for all to use. We have made the SEAL fitness program a major part of our mental and physical conditioning program."

—*John Cook*
1992 Olympic Volleyball Coach

This book is dedicated to all UDT/SEALs, past and present, who have perfected the meaning of perseverance and commitment.

And special thanks to my two children and family, who have been the inspiration behind this book with their love and support the entire way.

I also extend my gratitude to R. J. Wolf, without whose efforts this endeavor would not have been possible.

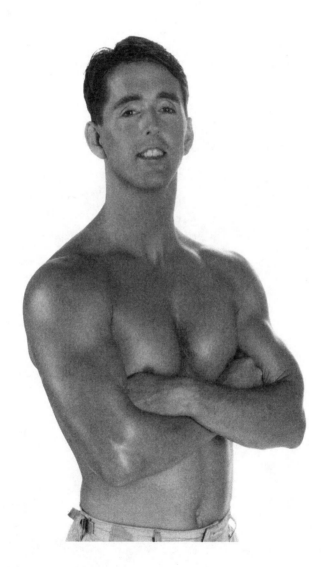

Contents

Introduction

Throughout the past decade the public has become increasingly aware of an elite group of individuals known as Navy SEALs. Without soliciting publicity, Navy SEALs have become recognized as some of the fittest people in the entire world. Today SEALs can be seen anywhere from *Muscle & Fitness* magazine to the Discovery channel on cable television.

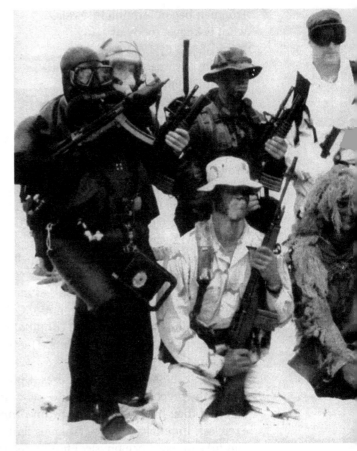

This training program will explain how these unique and dedicated people have achieved world prominence and an extraordinary reputation for physical fitness.

Resolve to stop thinking negative thoughts such as "I can't—there's too much for me to overcome," and start saying "I can! I will! Nobody will stop me!" Each day is a new day and a new start—so make yours happen with SEAL fitness.

Do not be fooled by the simplicity of the exercises you find in this book. Anybody can flip through these pages and say "This is it?" The key to this program's effectiveness is the format in which the exercises are performed (i.e., the pyramid system) and the complete blitzing of all muscle groups. If you are not sore after starting this program—or more accurately, if your muscles are not burning from exertion—you did not use the system properly.

SEAL HISTORY AND TRAINING

My purpose here is not to give you a complete and in-depth review of SEAL history but rather a basic understanding of who we are and where we come from. Also, you will better understand why it is paramount for us to excel in all areas of physical fitness and mental development.

In the early 1960s President John F. Kennedy, envisioning the path modern warfare was heading down, decided to organize an elite group of men specializing in counter-terrorist tactics. SEALs (an acronym for Sea, Air, Land) were selected from the ranks of the U.S. Navy's Underwater Demolition Teams (UDT).

SEALs have their roots in the Frogmen of World War II, who successfully performed covert amphibious missions against incredible odds. During the 1960s

Frogmen began forming into what is known today as Navy SEALs. By 1983 the term *UDT* was eliminated, and all UDT teams became SEAL teams.

Vietnam was the first arena for Navy SEALs to showcase their skills and prove their value as a combat unit. They proved their worth tenfold by becoming the most decorated unit and obtaining the highest kill-per-person ratio of any U.S. combat unit. SEALs were so feared by the Viet Cong that they were called "devils with green faces."

SEALs come from all walks of life—but that does not mean just *anyone* can be a Navy SEAL. You have to earn the right of passage. This is where BUD/S comes into the picture. BUD/S stands for Basic Underwater Demolition/SEAL School, which is located in Coronado, California. This is where all initial training for SEAL candidates is held. All candidates—officers and enlisted men alike— are required to pass the same tests. The training is excruciating and, for some, impossible.

BUD/S is broken into four phases. Upon arrival, you begin Preconditioning Phase. This is the preparatory phase, and the only phase where instructors can show a little bit of their human side. You begin running, swimming, and performing difficult exercises, improving your techniques daily. After an average of four to six weeks you take an entrance physical test to determine if you are ready to make the First Phase class.

Once the list of people who made it into the First Phase class is finalized, there is a traditional party on the beach the Saturday night before class begins. This is where all SEAL candidates shave their heads and celebrate wildly, because as of Monday, *life will end as they know it*. Starting Monday you will be property of the SEAL instructors.

First Phase is very demanding. The sixth week of First Phase is the infamous Hell Week. I'll explain more about that later. After Hell Week we were given one week in tennis shoes to allow the swelling in our feet to go down. Then we were right back in jungle boots. At that point we were qualified to learn SEAL tactics, stealth and concealment, and hydro reconnaissance.

Then came Second Phase, or Dive Phase. Here we learned about scuba diving with open-air scuba tanks. Once we gained the instructor's confidence, we were allowed to use pure-oxygen tanks.The stamina required for such grueling training was taking its toll, and the numbers in our class dwindled. We started out with a class of 130, and at this phase of training we were down to 75.

The Third Phase, Land Warfare, was spent half in Coronado and half on San Clemente Island. We learned about everything from land navigation and demolition tactics to small firearms.

We also had to increase our speed and endurance because the qualifying times for running and swimming were getting shorter and shorter. Even though our bodies were falling apart from the grueling training, we managed to keep up and pass the tests.

I'll never forget the feeling I had coming back from San Clemente Island knowing I only had one week of training left—walking tall and proud!

MY STORY

Having just gone through a divorce, I needed to get my head on straight and get some stability back into my life. I wanted to finish my college degree in marketing, but I was not in a financial position to cover the cost of college. Taking my father's recommendation I entered the Navy, hoping to utilize their college programs and complete my degree.

While at boot camp in San Diego, California, a recruiter came in and showed us a film about the SEAL program titled "Be Someone Special." My eyes lit up when I saw the training and skills required of a modern-day SEAL. I immediately knew that this was for me. Never one to sit behind a desk from nine to five, I just had to find out—to be pushed to my absolute limit. I kept asking myself if I could make it. My body was nearly 27 years old, and I had been out of shape since my football days in college six years ago. *Could I do it?*

I took the entrance exam and barely passed. Now I was really excited. I was going to get the electronics training (repairs of computers, radar, radios, etc.) I wanted, and I'd have the chance to become a Navy SEAL. Then, two weeks before graduation from boot camp, a counselor called me in and informed me that the electronics class was full, and that I would not be able to attend. Instead, I was offered three other classifications. I chose quartermaster.

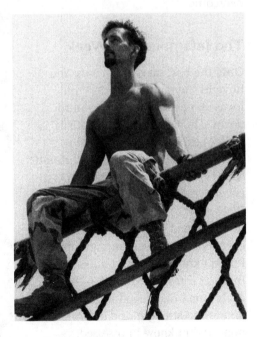

After graduating from boot camp as the top recruit, I was off to Orlando, Florida, for quartermaster training.

Once there, I was informed I had to take the entrance exam to BUD/s all over again! I was caught off guard—and as I later found out, this policy was only for Orlando. I was worried and started to panic because I had already lost the opportunity for electronics training and I didn't want to lose SEAL training as well. My entire career suddenly came down to one test that never should have been required. Have you ever been in that position?

Although I had stayed in good shape since boot camp, I had a feeling that my pull-ups were lacking. Sure enough, the day of the test I passed everything—except the pull-ups. While doing the last pull-up, the instructor told me to do just *one more* because I'd jerked my foot too much.

It all came down to that one last pull-up for me to qualify for SEAL training. *And I just couldn't do it!* I had nothing left in me, and my chin would not make it over the bar. I hopped off the bar in disbelief. My worst nightmare had come true—and my dreams were shattered. Then I became furious and told myself, "Mark, get off your rear and start working on your pull-ups. You will not let them beat you. You will not quit!" I had enough time for one more test before graduation from Quartermaster School. *Nothing* was going to stop me from passing the test this time!

Finally Judgment Day came! I passed the beginning portion of the test. Then it was time for pull-ups. Something sparked in me and I performed pull-up after pull-up without a problem. I did three more than required. I wanted to prove to the instructors that I had what it took to become a SEAL, to erase any doubt in their minds. I hopped off the bar and was silent. Then it hit me—I'm going to BUD/s! I soon graduated from the Orlando school in the top 5 percent of my class and was off to San Diego, California, for SEAL training.

In March 1991, when I arrived at BUD/s, it felt as though it were summer. I was immediately in love with San Diego. There are beautiful beaches everywhere, and the suburb of Coronado, where SEAL training is held, is like something straight out of a movie. Views throughout the city are breathtaking.

After I checked into BUD/s and received my basic gear, I began training in Fourth Phase. Every phase of BUD/s has its own unique tests and obstacles to overcome.

The Infamous Hell Week

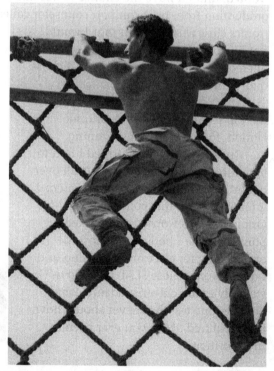

Only the best survive at BUD/s. You have to stay extremely alert and focused, never letting your guard down. The best example of this is Hell Week. This is the week that every BUD/s student must get through somehow—*some way*—if he wants to become a Navy SEAL. During Hell Week, every training scenario you have learned up to that point is executed. There were many times I didn't know if I would make it through a test or evaluation, but each time I dug deep inside myself and found strength and determination I didn't know I possessed.

Throughout the entire week you only get a half-hour of sleep, here and there, and never more than two hours total. The majority of the time you are soaking wet—either from hoses or surf torture. Surf torture is where you have to get in the ocean's surf zone and let the waves crash down on your face. The extensive amount of time we had to spend in the surf zone brought us dangerously close to hypothermia, and many SEAL candidates were disqualified during this exercise. Somehow I made it through Hell Week—taking one day at a time, and not looking too far into the future.

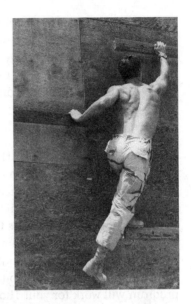

Once through Hell Week and First Phase, I was ready for Dive Phase (Second Phase) and Land Warfare (Third Phase). After completing both, an unbelievable dream came true—BUD/s graduation! Phase by phase I had gotten through and made new friends and bonds that would last a lifetime.

It was a very emotional time for me; I was so proud of myself. Many people close to me doubted I could achieve my goal, but I refused to let anyone stop me. I was 28 years old, in the best shape of my life—faster and stronger than I had been when I was 18—and I'd just accomplished what guys six to eight years younger than me had done.

My next assignment was SEAL Team Three. And the dream continued!

YOU CAN DO IT!

Many people believe the only way to get in shape is by putting a lot of money into trendy fitness centers, or spending hard-earned cash on a variety of workout videotapes. In the end, these methods seldom provide the results we're all looking for. But don't get me wrong—I am not demeaning gyms or workout tapes; in fact, I still enjoy the benefits of a gym to keep fit. Weight-lifting rooms and other facilities can be extremely beneficial. However, to obtain and maintain supreme cardiovascular fitness and a rock-hard body, I must continually use the training regimen I learned as a member of the Navy SEALs.

You will find that I use the word *results* quite often. Isn't that what we are looking for? This program was not developed to motivate you. I will not give you any false hopes. This program is for someone who is already motivated to seek the ultimate level of fitness! I will not guarantee 100 percent results. No program can truthfully guarantee 100 percent results because everyone has a different level of motivation and potential. If anyone guarantees you 100 percent results, then they are trying to deceive you. However, I can tell you from painful personal experience that results can only come from dedication and deep desire within yourself. If you are tired of being out of shape, or if you're seeking an incredible challenge—then use this program and watch your body reach fitness levels you never dreamed possible. There's no denying the effects it had on me.

No one can deny the Navy SEALs' reputation in fitness is second to none. I've seen people lose 20 pounds in one month and their fitness levels skyrocket using these exact same exercises that you too can perform in your own backyard.

The Mental Edge

SEALs are frequently asked, "How were you able to make it through such torturous training?" The most common answer is "I was mentally tough!" In addition to superior athletic ability and physical fitness, one thing all SEALs have in common that enables them to survive training is *determination*. The central driving force of success is in your own mind, which is the key to all of your strength and motivation. If you want results from this program, start by strengthening yourself *mentally*.

The biggest impression that SEAL training has left on me is that the human body will perform beyond limits you never thought possible to achieve. Never doubt this program will work for you! Thousands of SEALs, past and present, can testify that it does work!

Here are some tips to help you get started.

- **First, be determined to succeed.** Clearly identify the fitness results you want—and vow to yourself that no individual or obstacle is going to stop you from achieving your goal. A goal not written is just a dream. Once you've written down your goal, it is more than just a dream—it's a clearly defined objective. Create long-term and short-term goals. Write down your long-term goals, then set short-term or smaller goals to achieve your ultimate goal. By concentrating on and accomplishing your short-term goals, you will achieve your long-term goals.
- **Review your goals often to stay motivated.** Keep your list of goals in a highly visible place, so you can read them often and stay motivated. With this attitude you will be ready to achieve a rock-hard body in an incredibly short amount of time.
- **Make a visual record of your progress.** Take a picture of yourself before you start this program and every three months thereafter, so you can visually monitor your progress. You are going to be so

amazed! Determine in your mind what you want to look like and don't compromise. With this program, your goals can be reached. Record your desired weight, measurements, and endurance levels through each phase. (For your convenience, forms to record your progress are included in Chapter 9 of this book.)

- **Above all, remember this:** I did it—and so can you.

Now get busy!

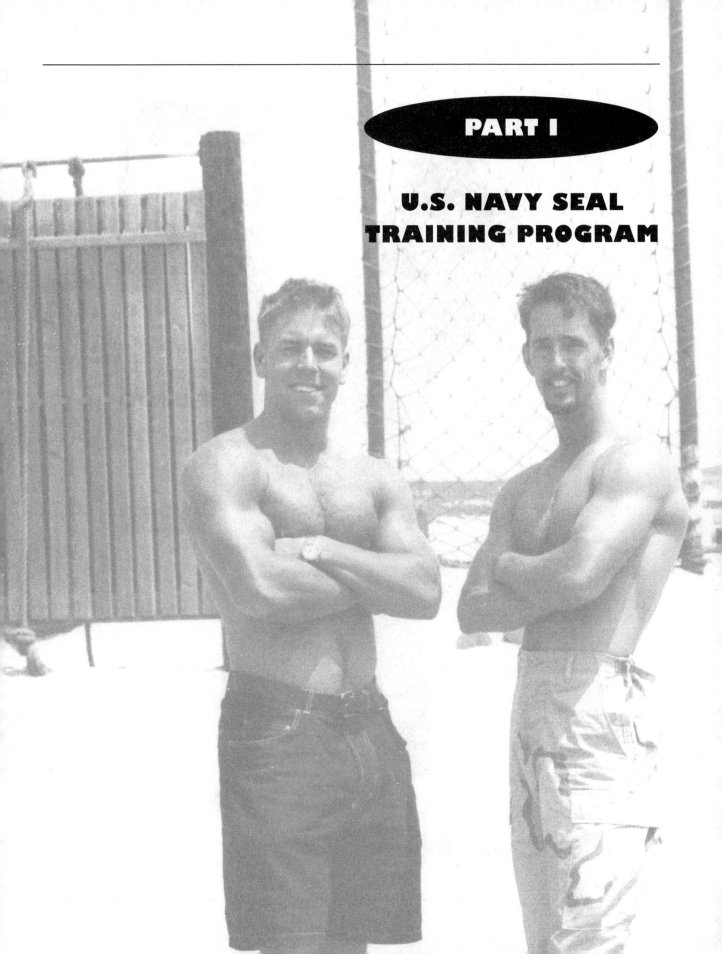

PART I

U.S. NAVY SEAL
TRAINING PROGRAM

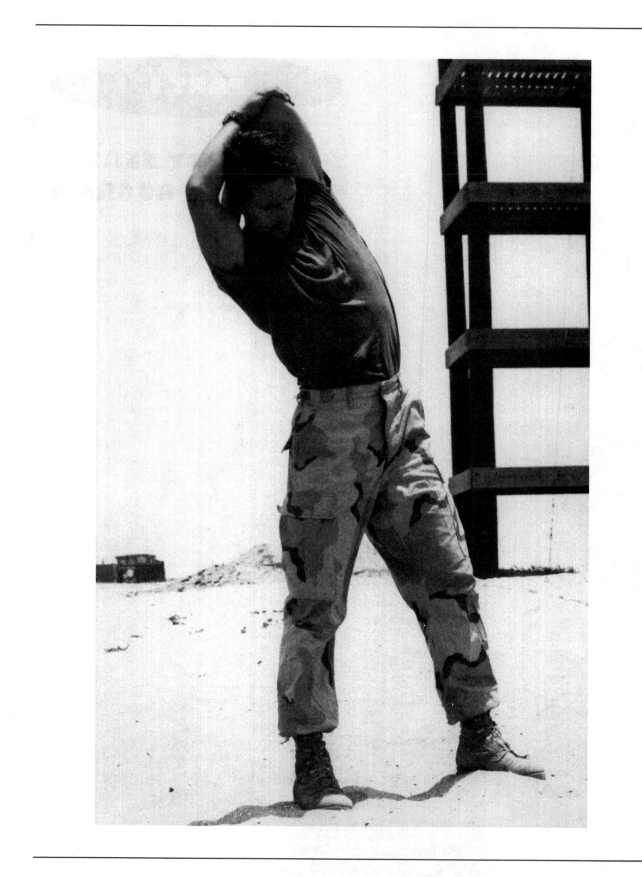

1. Stretching

Stretching can be one of the most neglected areas of a workout. I cannot stress the importance of stretching enough. As a Navy SEAL, I could not perform at the peak levels expected of me without first warming up my body. Due to stiffness or a lack of motion, joints, tendons, ligaments, and muscles can easily tear. By stretching, we allow ourselves a greater range of motion, which in turn prevents injuries.

You will achieve your best range of motion and flexibility if your muscles are lightly worked before stretching. Not so long ago it was commonly thought that the key to effective flexibility was stretching while your muscles were cold, *before* any activity. It is now known that stretching cold muscles is *not* the most efficient method.

Before actually stretching, it is best to start with two to five minutes of jumping jacks and push-ups to warm up the upper body, and/or five minutes of light jogging or bicycle riding to warm the legs. This gets the blood flowing into the muscles and makes them more pliable and able to stretch, preparing them for a more effective stretching session. Once this step is finished, and only when you feel warm, begin stretching.

Throughout these stretches remember to proceed *slowly*. Try to hold each stretch for at least 15 seconds—and *never* bounce! You should feel pulling, not pain. Pulling can be described as a gradual discomfort or slight soreness due to tight muscles. As you stretch longer, tightness will decrease and flexibility will increase. Pain can be described as a sharp, intense sensation causing great discomfort to a specific body part. This can happen when you do not stretch slowly. As you continue your daily stretching you will be able to distinguish pulling from pain and recognize how to loosen your muscles.

Using the stretches I have listed here, your total preworkout stretching time should be approximately 15 minutes. When your workout is completed, do at least 10 more minutes of stretching. This is when you will be most limber and when you'll achieve the greatest gain in flexibility. It is important to stretch not only before and after exercising, but also *during* the exercise program. While you are working out, your muscle fibers begin to tighten. By stretching during your workout you loosen up muscle fibers, allowing more fibers to be affected—which allows for much greater results.

UPPER BODY STRETCHES
1. Upper Body Stretch

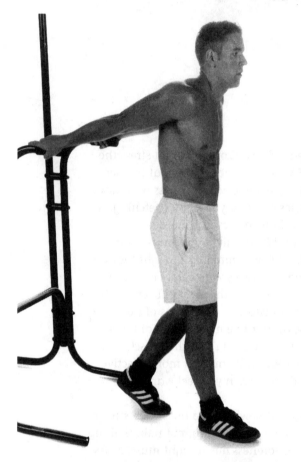

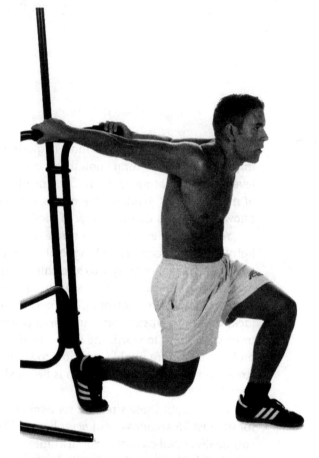

FIGURE 1	FIGURE 2

- Find something you can grab onto with both hands, at about chest level.
- Place both arms behind you and grab the object, palms down.

- Lean forward, then to the right, and then to the left.
- Lean as far as you can each way.
- Concentrate on stretching your chest and your arms.
- To get the best stretch possible, do this exercise *slowly*.

2. Single Arm Stretch

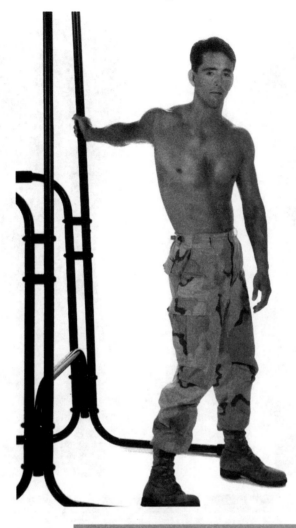

FIGURE 1

- Find something you can grab onto with both hands, at about chest level.
- Place one arm behind you and grab this object, palm out and away.
- Stretch only one arm at a time. Isolating each side increases the effectiveness of the stretch.
- Muscle flexibility will enable you to perform a greater number of repetitions. The more repetitions you perform, the more you'll increase your muscle strength and development.
- To get the best stretch possible, do this exercise *slowly*.

3. Triceps Stretch

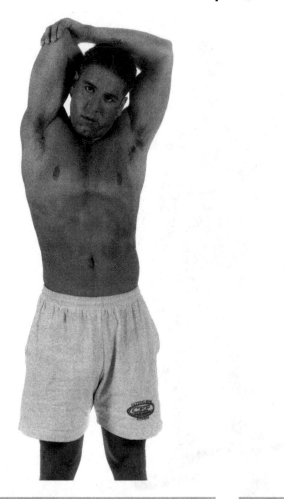

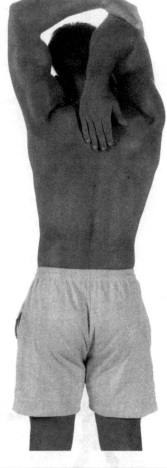

FIGURE 1

Place your right hand behind your head and down the middle of your back, as far as it will go.

FIGURE 2

Now place your left hand on your right elbow and begin stretching toward your left.

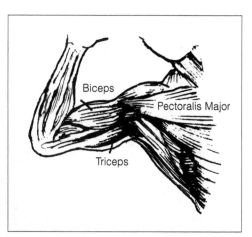

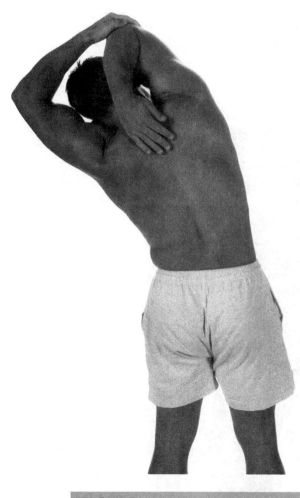

FIGURE 3

- Once you reach the *discomfort zone*, maintain that position for 15 to 30 seconds.
- Switch sides and repeat.

4. Shoulder Stretch

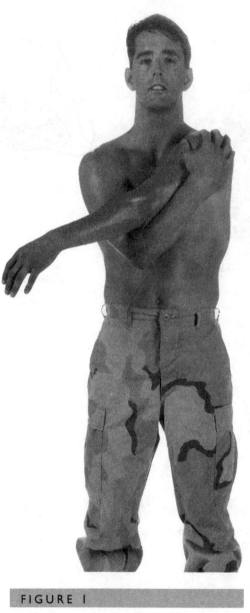

FIGURE 1

- Bring your right arm across your chest.
- Place your right elbow in the inside joint of your left arm, then reach across and grab your left shoulder.

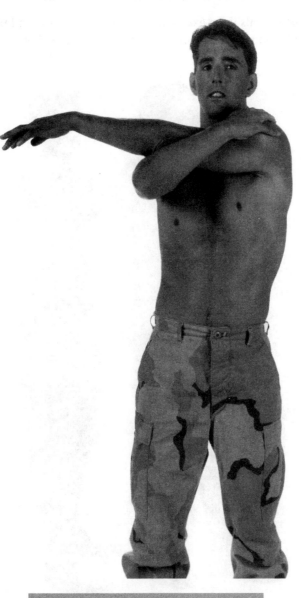

FIGURE 2

- Squeeze and elevate your right elbow.
- Hold this position for 15 to 30 seconds, then release.
- Switch sides and repeat.

5. Two-Person Chest Stretch

If you have a partner, this is an excellent stretch for the chest and biceps. Main emphasis should be on you. Arms should not be forced together.

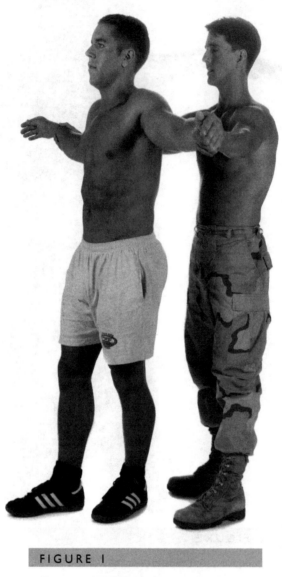

FIGURE 1

- Place your hands behind you with your thumbs up, palms facing out.
- Behind you, your partner places his hands on your wrists.

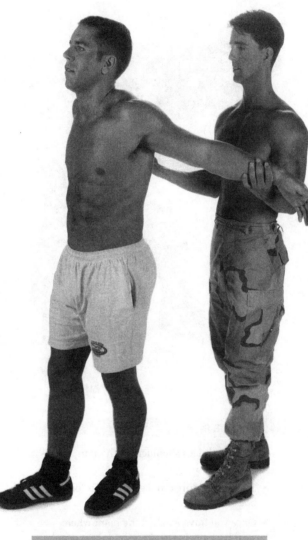

FIGURE 2

- Your partner carefully brings your wrists back as close together as possible.

- Hold this position for 15 seconds, then release.

6. Fore and Aft Stretch

This one will help stretch your abs and your lower back. To prevent added stress to the back, it is important to keep your back straight while bending over with your knees slightly bent. This is a good stretch to perform before and after the ab routine.

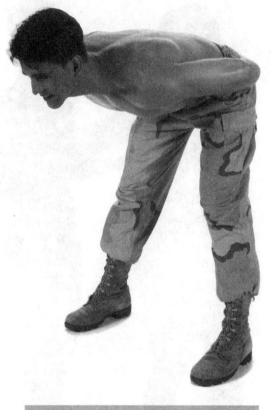

FIGURE 1

- Stand with legs shoulder-width apart, hands on your hips.

- Slowly bend forward, keeping your lower back straight.

- Once you have reached the point where your back begins to get tight, take a deep breath and, as you exhale, try stretching a little more.

- Hold this position for 15 seconds, then release.

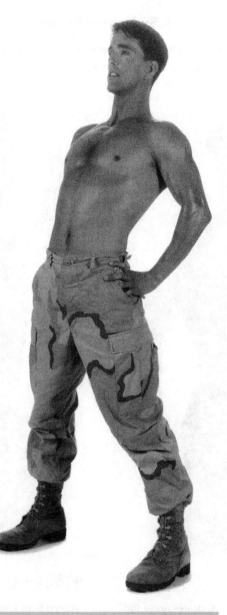

FIGURE 2

- Now lean back, pushing your hips until your stomach is tight.
- Hold this position for 15 seconds, then release.

7. Swimmer Stretch

This is a good stretch for the chest and anterior deltoids. It can be used before and after the push-up segment. Perform this stretch *slowly*.

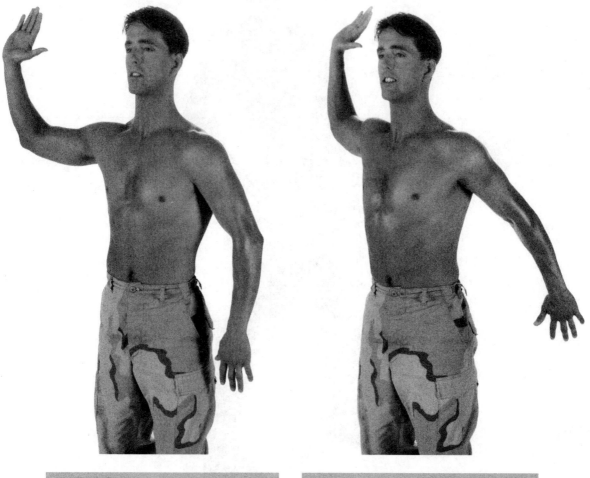

FIGURE 1

Hold your right hand at a 90-degree angle facing upward and your left hand at a 90-degree angle facing downward.

FIGURE 2

- Stretch both hands backward at the same time until your chest is tight.

- Release; return to the original position.

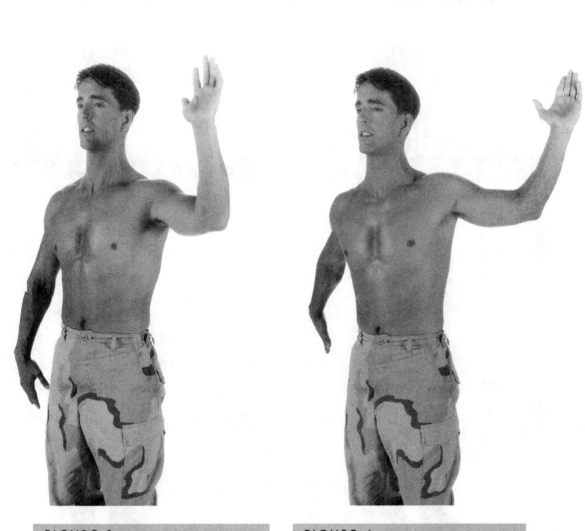

FIGURE 3

Place your left hand at a 90-degree angle facing upward and your right hand at a 90-degree angle facing downward.

FIGURE 4

- Stretch both hands backward at the same time until your chest is tight.
- Release; return to the original position.

8. Press/Press-Fling

This is a good chest stretch that can be used before and after the push-up segment.

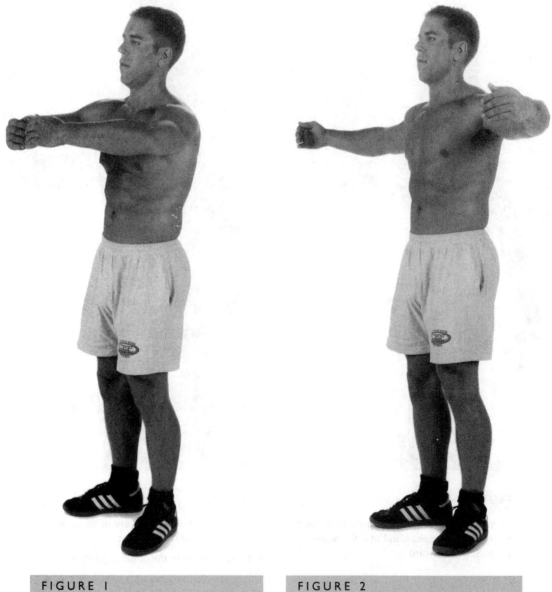

FIGURE 1

Bring your hands in front of your chest, palms facing inward.

FIGURE 2

- In one fluid motion, extend your hands and arms outward but no farther than shown above.

- Maintain hands and arms in a half-circle configuration through the movement.

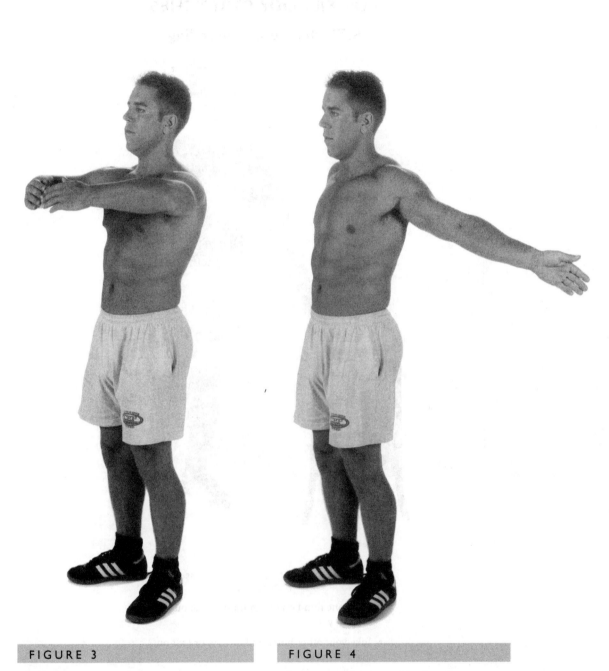

FIGURE 3

Bring your hands and arms back to the original position shown in Figure 1.

FIGURE 4

Extend your arms out and back as far as possible, but release your hands at the very end of the motion so that your arms are completely straight.

LOWER BODY STRETCHES

9. Thigh Stretch—Standing

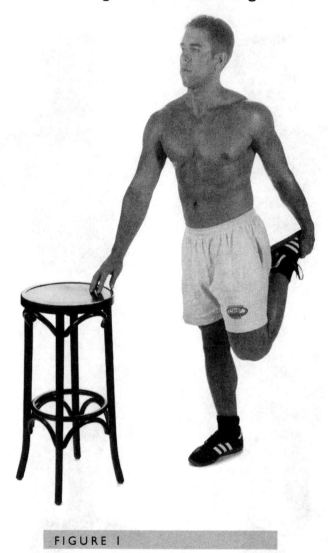

FIGURE I

- Place one hand on anything stable enough to support you.

- Take your other hand and grab your foot on the same side.

FIGURE 2

- Pull your foot up behind you, stretching your thigh.
- Switch sides and repeat.

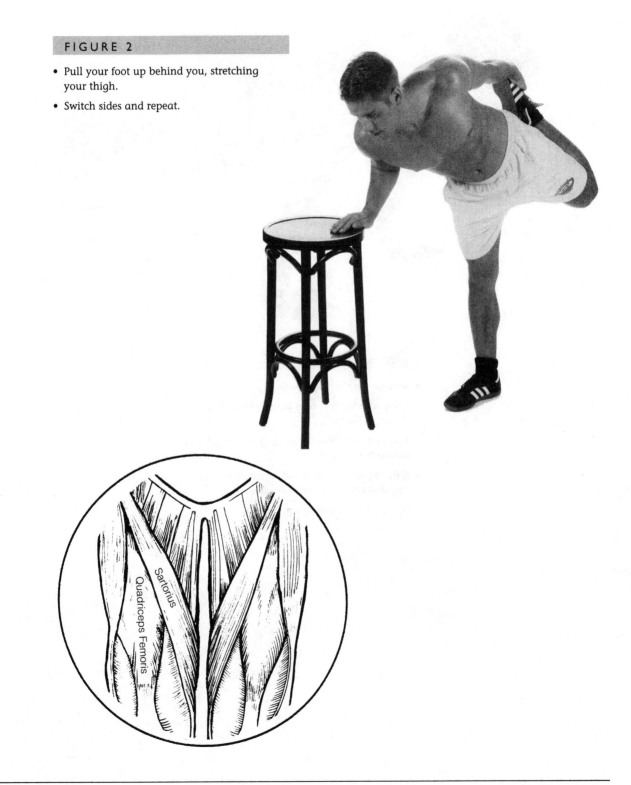

10. Calf Stretch

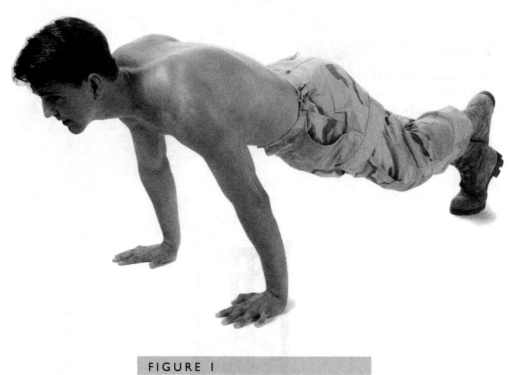

FIGURE 1

- Assume the push-up position.
- Place your left foot over your right heel, as shown in Figure 2.
- Taking it very slow, try placing your right heel flat on the ground.
- If the tightness in your calf becomes painful, stop and ease up on the pressure.
- Switch to the other leg and repeat.

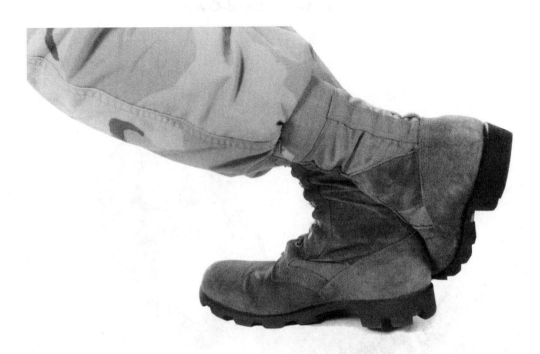

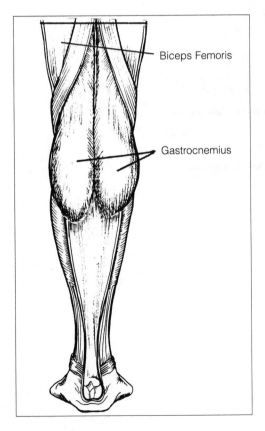

Biceps Femoris

Gastrocnemius

FIGURE 2

Your feet should be in this position.

11. Sit-Down Bend-Over

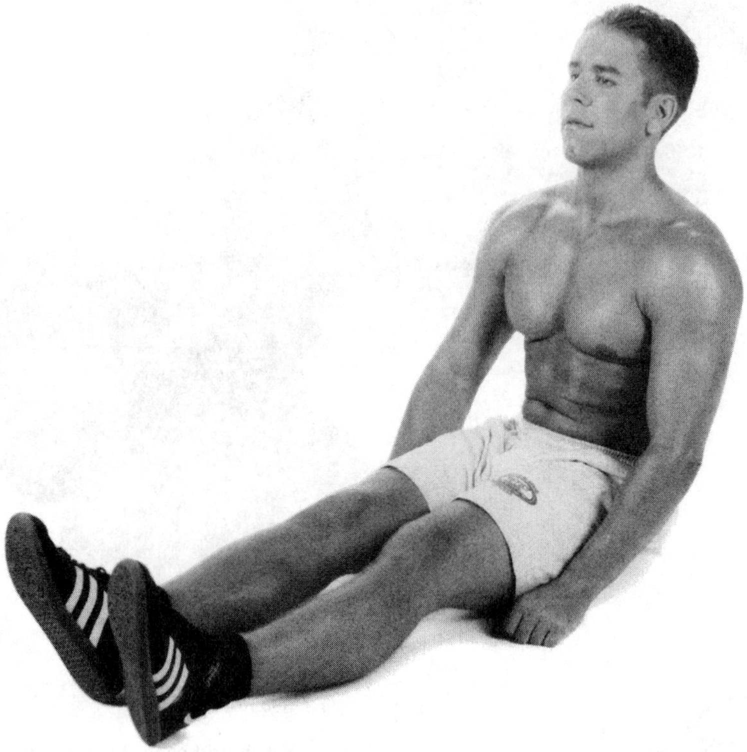

FIGURE 1

- Sit on the ground. Keep your legs together.
- The key factor is to keep your legs straight, with a slight bend in your knees.
- Maintain a straight back throughout the stretch.

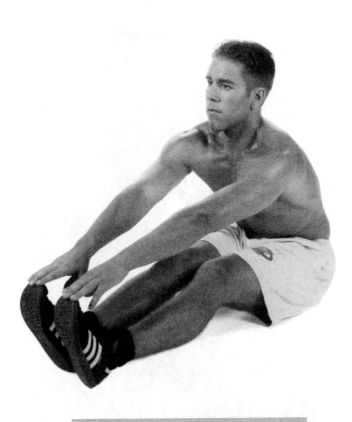

FIGURE 2

- Lean over and try to touch your toes with your hands.

- Hold for 10 to 15 seconds, then release.

12. Hurdler's Stretch

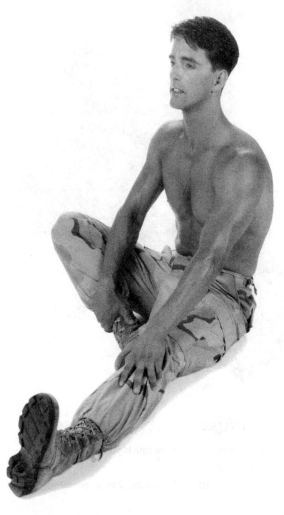

FIGURE 1

- Sit down.
- Bend your right leg inward, so that your foot is flat against the inside of your left knee or thigh.
- Place your right hand on your right foot (or your right ankle, depending on which position is most comfortable for you).

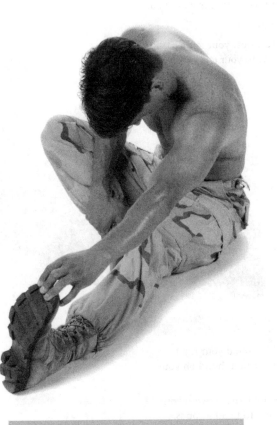

FIGURE 2

- Lean over toward your left foot. Try to touch your chest to your knee.

- Switch legs and repeat.

13. ITB Stretch

This stretch is great for loosening a tight lower back and for stretching the ITB (iliotibial) tendon, which runs from your hip to your knee.

FIGURE 1

- Sit down with your legs out in front of you.
- Keep your left leg straight.
- Cross your right foot over your left leg and place your foot next to your left knee.

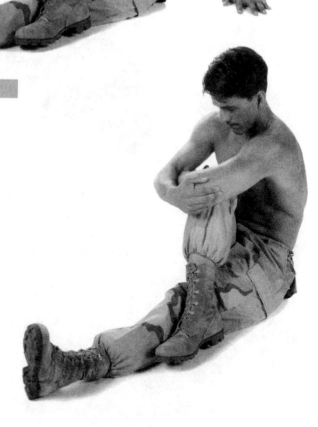

FIGURE 2

- Wrap your left arm around your right knee, then place your right hand on your left elbow.
- Slowly bring your right knee toward your chest, and hold it for 15 to 30 seconds, then release.

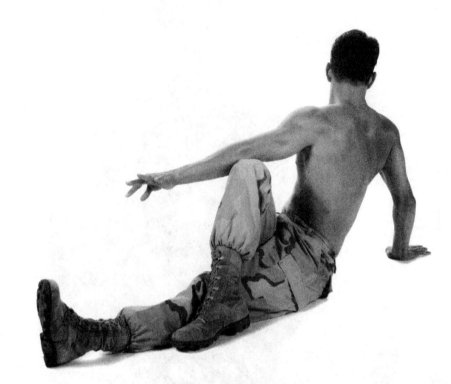

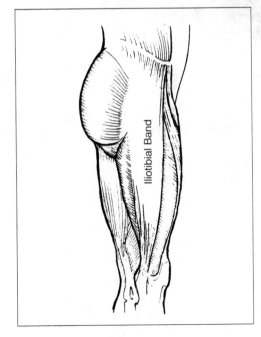

Iliotibial Band

FIGURE 3

- Next, place the outer part of your left elbow against the outer part of your right knee while reaching back with your right hand.

- Place your right hand on the ground about a foot behind your lower back.

- Slowly twist to the right while pushing your right knee to the left.

- Hold this position 15 seconds, then release.

- Switch to the other leg and repeat.

14. Butterfly Stretch

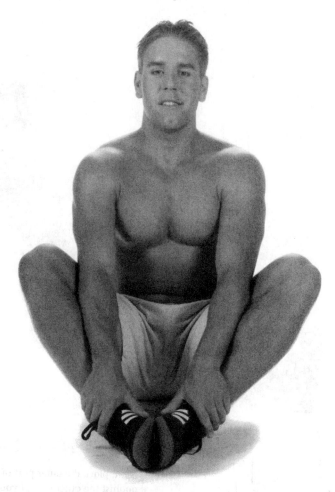

FIGURE 1

- Sit down.
- Place your heels together to make a diamond shape with your legs.
- Grab your ankles and slowly bring your heels toward you until they are about six inches from your crotch.

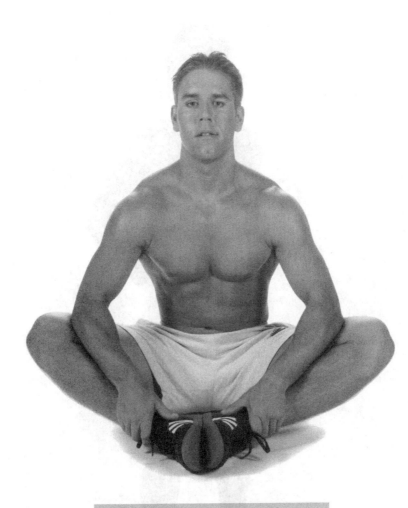

FIGURE 2

- Put pressure on your knees by placing your elbows on the inside of your knees and pushing downward.

- Hold this position for 15 seconds.

- Release and relax for 10 seconds.

- Repeat the process again, three to four times.

15. Trunk Extensions

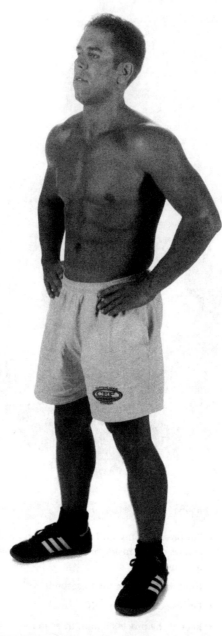

FIGURE 1

- Stand up straight, with your feet shoulder-width apart.

- Place your hands on your waist.

- Keep your legs straight.

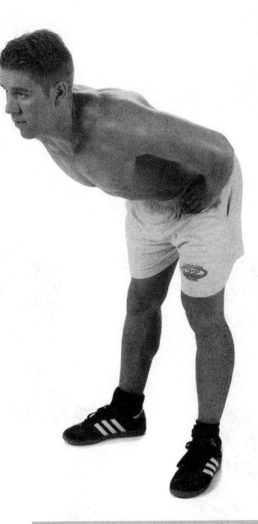

FIGURE 2

- Lean forward as far as you can; hold for 15 seconds.

- Straighten back up.

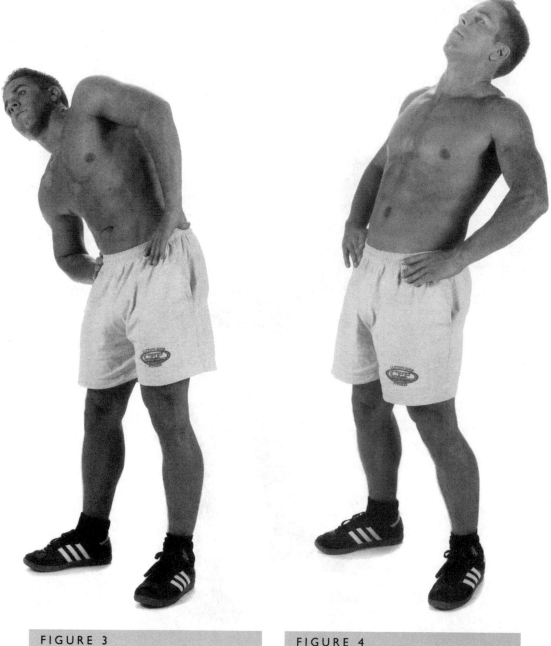

FIGURE 3

- Now lean to your right side.
- Hold for 15 seconds.

FIGURE 4

- Lean to the back, thrust your hips forward and keep your hands on your waist.
- Hold for 15 seconds.

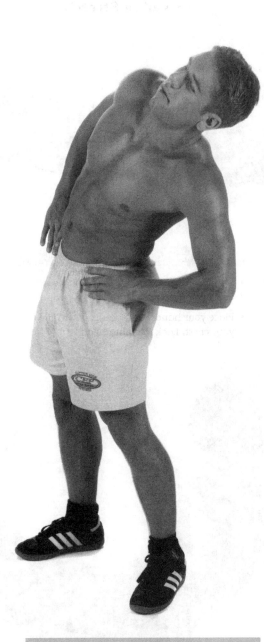

FIGURE 5

- Now lean to your left side.
- Hold for 15 seconds, then release.

Keep your knees bent to prevent hyperextending your back. This first repetition should be slow. Following repetitions can be more fluid. You will soon be able to rotate smoothly through each phase of this exercise.

16. Cobra Stretch

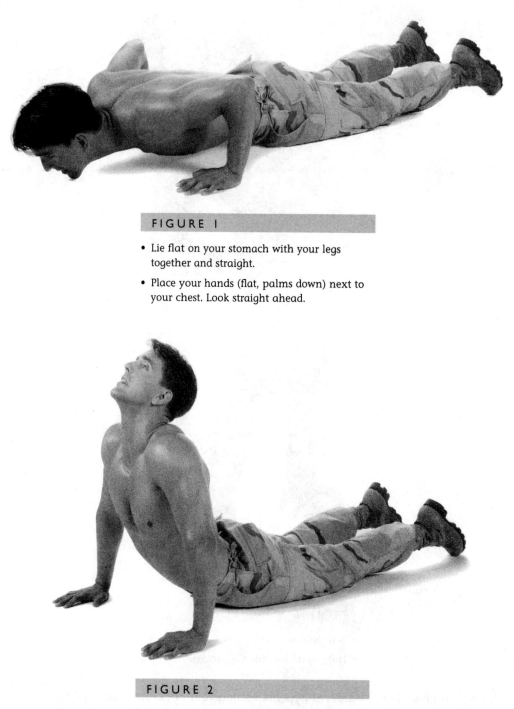

FIGURE 1

- Lie flat on your stomach with your legs together and straight.
- Place your hands (flat, palms down) next to your chest. Look straight ahead.

FIGURE 2

Raise your upper torso and roll your head back.

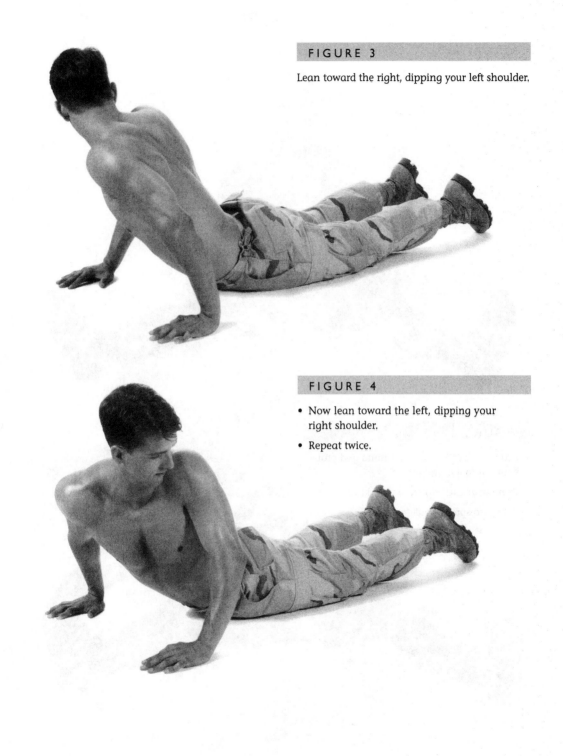

FIGURE 3

Lean toward the right, dipping your left shoulder.

FIGURE 4

- Now lean toward the left, dipping your right shoulder.
- Repeat twice.

17. Hamstring Stretch

FIGURE 1

Assume a spread-eagle position.

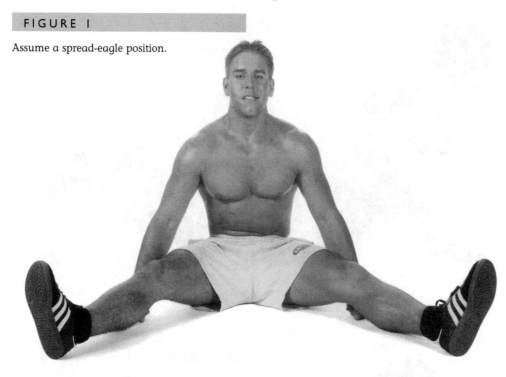

FIGURE 2

- Reach over with your right hand and grab your left foot or ankle.
- Bring your chest down to your knee.
- Return to spread-eagle position.

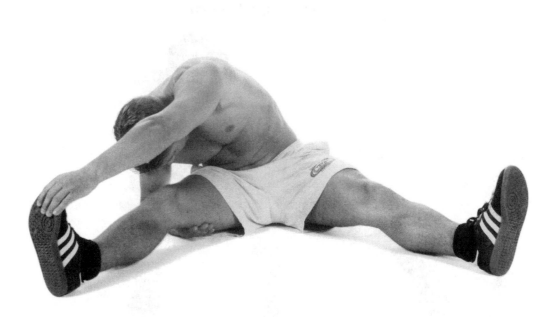

FIGURE 3

- Reach over with your left hand and grab your right foot.
- Bring your chest down to your knee.

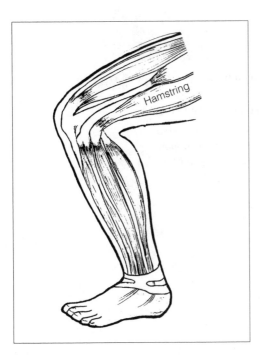

18. Inner-Thigh Stretch

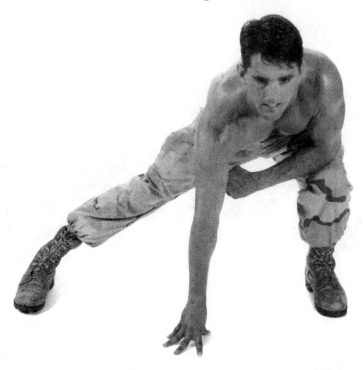

FIGURE 1

- Place your right hand on the ground for support.

- Extend your right foot and leg out to the side.

- Lean toward your left knee while placing your left elbow on your thigh for support. Do not allow your left knee to go past a 90-degree angle.

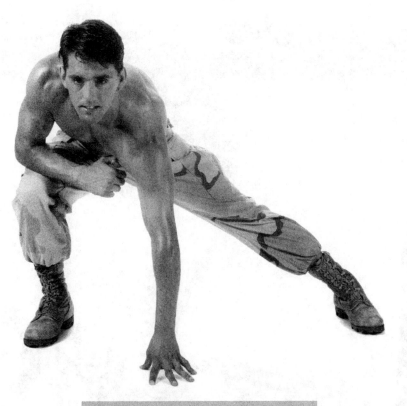

FIGURE 2

- Place your left hand on the ground for support.

- Extend your left foot and leg out to the side.

- Lean toward your knee while placing your right elbow on your thigh for support. Do not allow your left knee to go past a 90-degree angle.

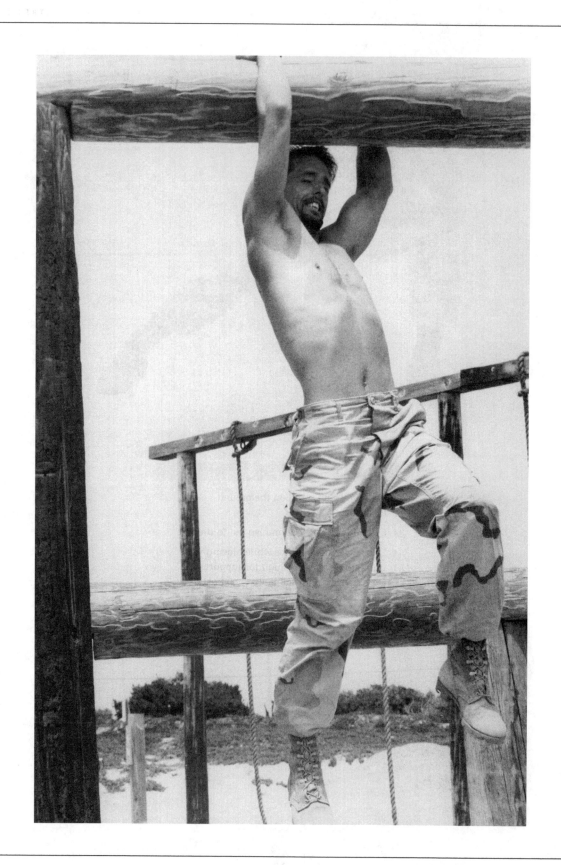

2. Upper Body Workout

The upper body is the area where, not counting your abdominals, you will see the quickest results. Just as you stretch during the stomach and leg exercises, it is extremely important to stretch *throughout* your upper body routine. Using the upper body stretches I've shown you will allow you to pump out more repetitions.

I have divided the upper body workout into three sections because of the rate of growth and changes these muscles go through. For maximum benefit, do the exercises in the order I have written them. This order will "burn out" your upper body before the push-ups, which will lead to a more effective push-up session. The upper body workout utilizes the pyramid system (ascending repetitions, followed by corresponding descending repetitions). As an example, let's go through the Upper Body Workout—Beginner Program for week one (page 66).

1. First, do 1 regular pull-up. Drop off the pull-up bar. Rest 15 seconds.
2. Next, do 2 regular pull-ups. Drop off the pull-up bar. Rest 15 seconds. Then do 1 more pull-up, drop off the bar, and rest 15 seconds.
3. Now do the reverse-grip pull-up, utilizing the same system.

After you have finished the pull-ups, move to the bar dips. Do 4 sets of 5 dips, with a 15- to 30-second rest in between sets. Move on to the push-ups. Do 2 regular push-ups. Rest 15 seconds. Do 4 more regular push-ups. Rest 15 seconds. Do 2 more regular push-ups. Rest 15 seconds.

Now move to the triceps push-ups (page 60) utilizing the same format for these and the rest of the push-ups.

Do not—I repeat: *do not*—sacrifice form for repetition. Just because you are one repetition away from finally reaching the advanced level does not mean you may break form and raise your buttocks into the air, or fail to touch your chest on the ground. Do not cheat yourself. You have plenty of time.

WHEN TO ADVANCE

You do not have to reach the next level in all exercises before advancing. If you can perform intermediate-level push-ups but only beginning-level pull-ups, that's fine.

Always do as much as you can without injuring yourself. The average person will advance faster in push-ups and bar dips than in pull-ups. It all depends on each person's individual strength and fitness level.

Continually strive to increase your repetitions. After the first week, increase your push-ups. By the fifth week you should be doing four sets of eight dips. Once you reach your fifth week, you will be able to increase your repetitions weekly. This will become quite challenging. And don't forget—your greatest gain in fitness and strength will occur when you use proper form.

It's time to go to work.

Good luck!

19. Regular Pull-Up

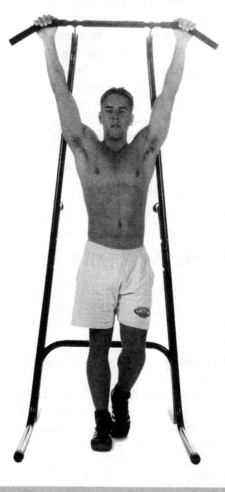

FIGURE 1

This exercise can only be performed on a secure pull-up bar. Grasp the pull-up bar so that your hands are shoulder-width apart.

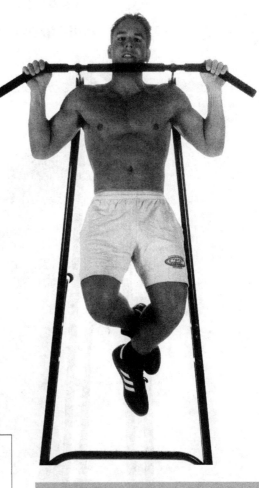

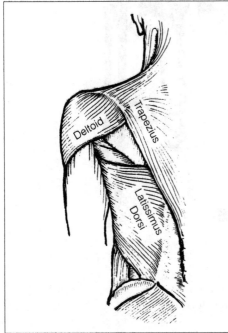

FIGURE 2

- Raise your body up so that your chin is at or above the level of the pull-up bar.

- Lower your body slowly to prevent injury.

- When you are fully extended down, start back up again.

TRAINING TIP
Pull-Up (by Yourself)

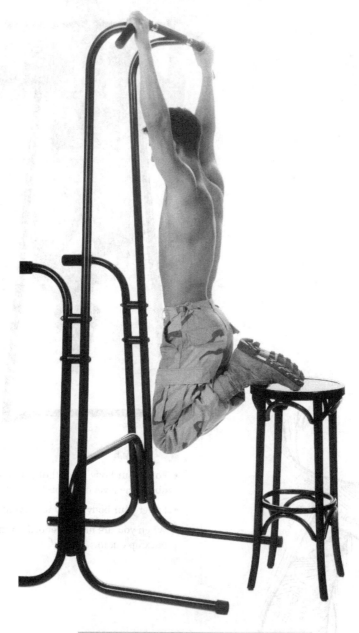

Take an ordinary stool and place it below you, so that you can rest your feet on top. Do not use the stool to support you; it is just a balancing tool.

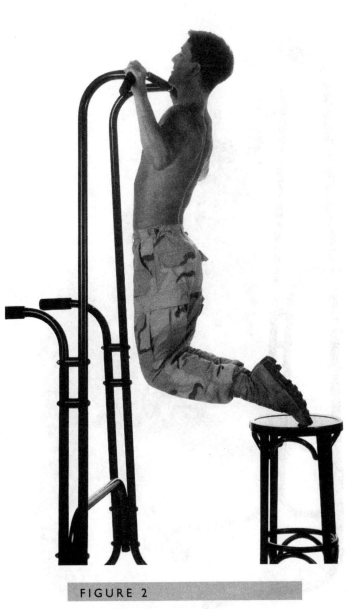

FIGURE 2

- Use only your thigh muscles to elevate your upper body.

- Just remember to release your feet before dropping off the pull-up bar—or else landing will be a very unpleasant experience.

TRAINING TIP

Pull-Up (with a Partner)

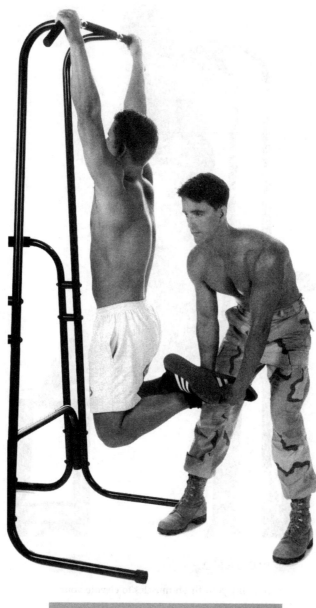

FIGURE 1

This photograph demonstrates the proper pull-up technique.

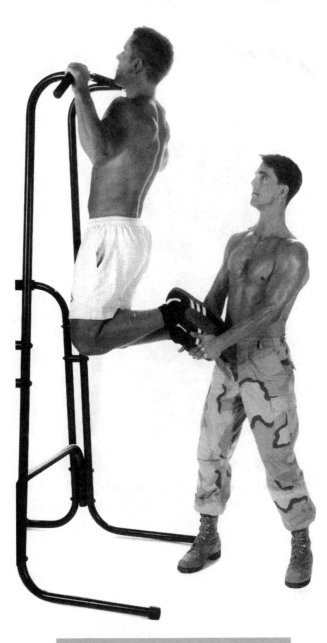

FIGURE 2

The key to this technique is to have your partner hold your feet steady at a 90-degree angle
while you use your thigh muscles to elevate
your body.

20. Reverse-Grip Pull-Up

This exercise will work your biceps and upper back.

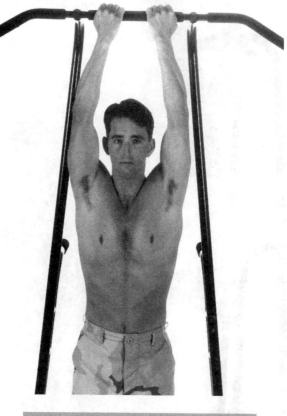

FIGURE I

Place your hands on the pull-up bar as shown
(2 to 3 inches apart), palms facing you.

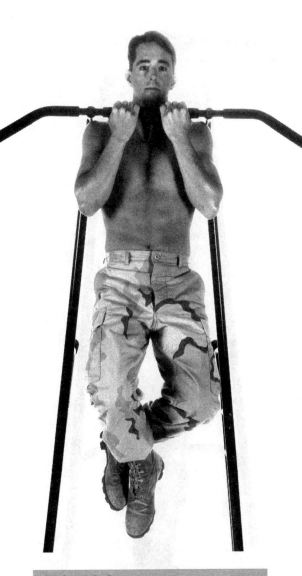

FIGURE 2

- Pull yourself up until your chin is above the bar.
- Lower yourself down slowly, then start back up again.

21. Close-Grip Pull-Up

This exercise will work your forearms, triceps, and upper back.

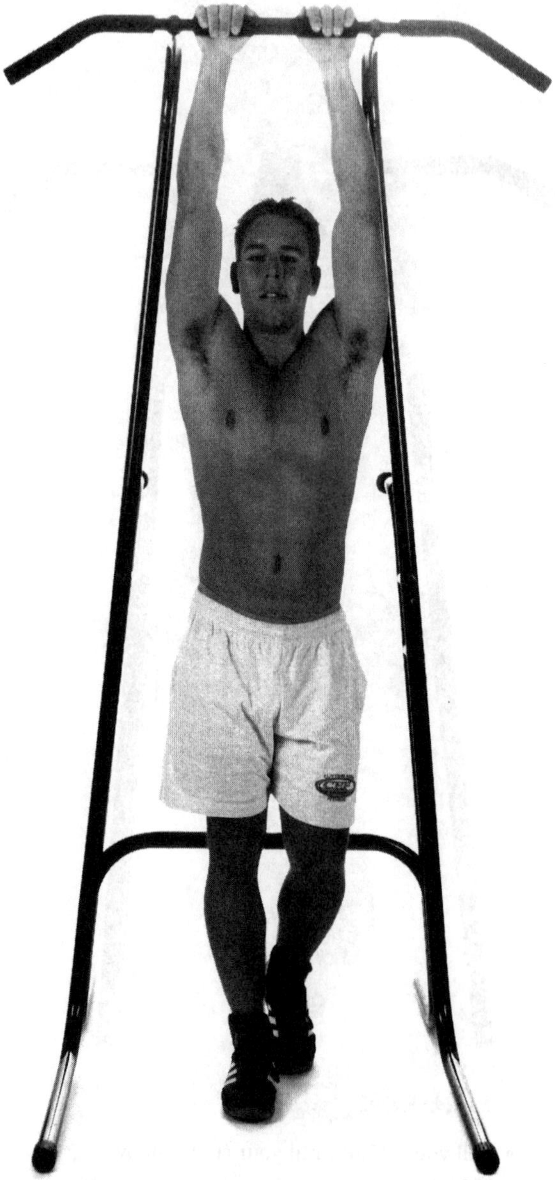

FIGURE I

Place your hands on the pull-up bar, as shown (2 to 3 inches apart), with your palms facing away from you.

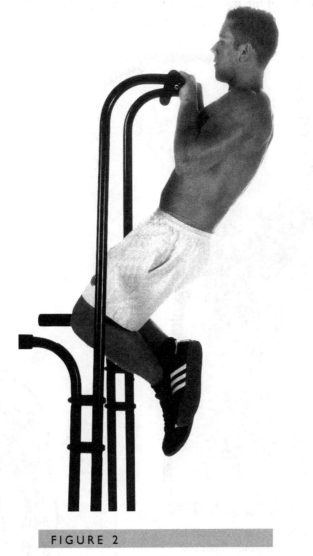

FIGURE 2

- Pull yourself up so that your chin is above the bar.

- Lower your body *slowly* to prevent injury.

- When you are fully extended down, start back up again.

22. Behind-the-Neck Pull-Up

This is an incredible exercise for the upper middle back and lats. You'll notice that every Navy SEAL has incredible back development. This exercise is a major reason why. This is also one of the most difficult exercises to perform.

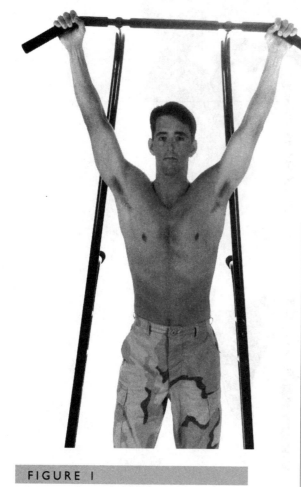

FIGURE 1

Place your hands on the bar, just past shoulder width, with your palms facing away from you.

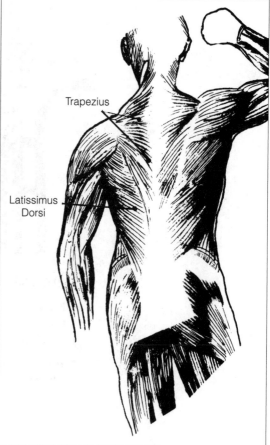

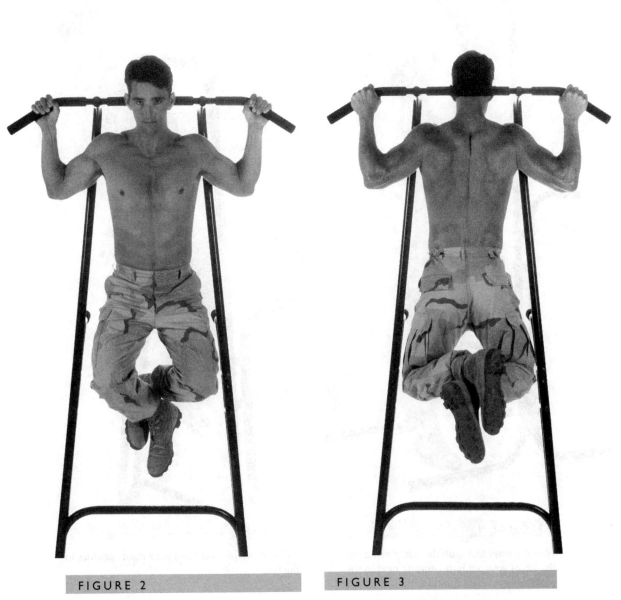

FIGURE 2

Raise yourself up . . .

FIGURE 3

. . . but instead of placing your chin above the bar, make the bar touch the back of your neck, as close to your shoulders as possible.

23. Commando Pull-Up

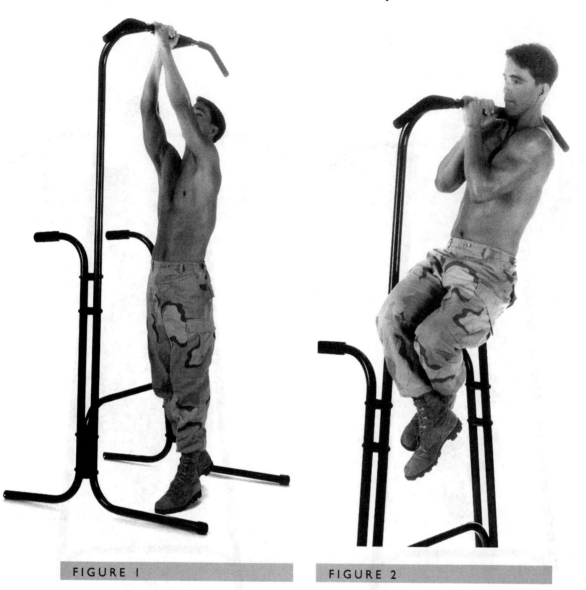

Face sideways and grab the bar, placing the thumb of your left hand directly next to the pinkie of your right hand . . .

Pull yourself up, touching your right shoulder to the bar.

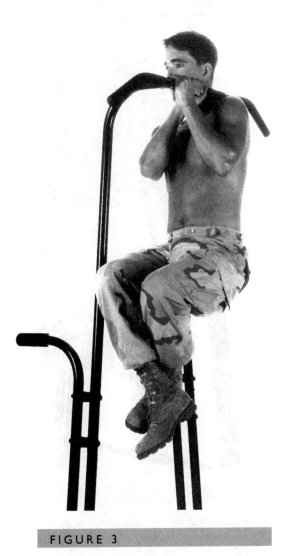

FIGURE 3

- Lower yourself down slowly, then pull yourself back up again, so the bar touches your left shoulder. That counts as one repetition.

- Do not jerk yourself up during this or any pull-up exercise since that will not isolate any muscle group. Jerking yourself up relies too much on your body's momentum, rather than on muscle performance.

24. Bar Dip

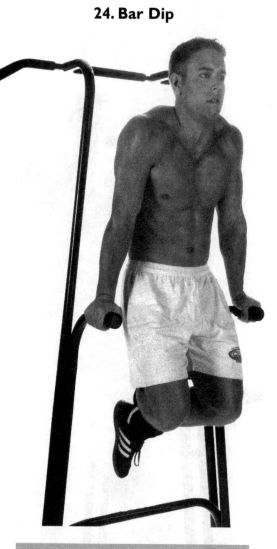

FIGURE I

Place your hands on two solid objects or bars
placed shoulder-width apart.

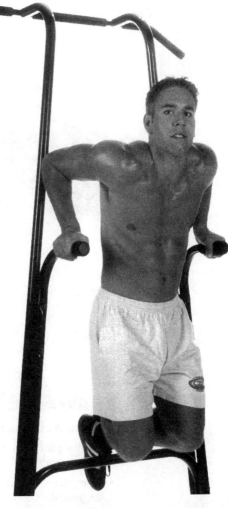

FIGURE 2

- Lower yourself until your elbows are bent at a 90-degree angle.
- Push yourself back until your arms are straight again, as shown in Figure 1.

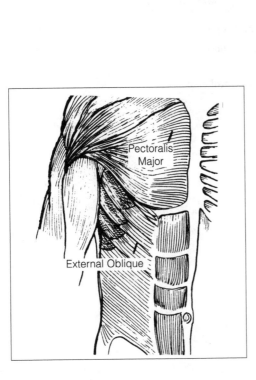

Pectoralis Major

External Oblique

25. Push-Up

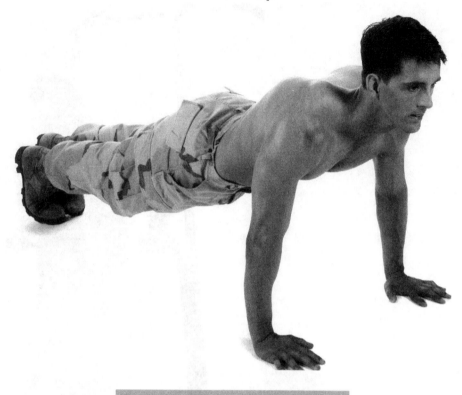

FIGURE 1

- Assume the standard push-up position.
- Position your arms slightly beyond shoulder width.
- Keep your body perfectly parallel to the ground.

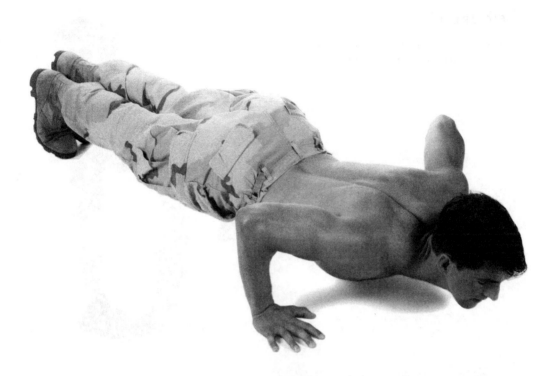

FIGURE 2

- Bend your elbows and lower yourself until your chest (lightly) touches the ground.

- Immediately push yourself back up to the starting position.

- Fully extend your arms when coming back up.

Remember: no cheating!

Do not rest your chest on the ground! During SEAL training that was a *big* mistake! If you tried to rest your chest on the ground, or if you were not going all the way down, the instructor would make you stop and start all over again—which often resulted in triple the original number!

26. Triceps Push-Up

FIGURE 1

This is similar to a regular push-up except that you spread your feet shoulder-width apart.

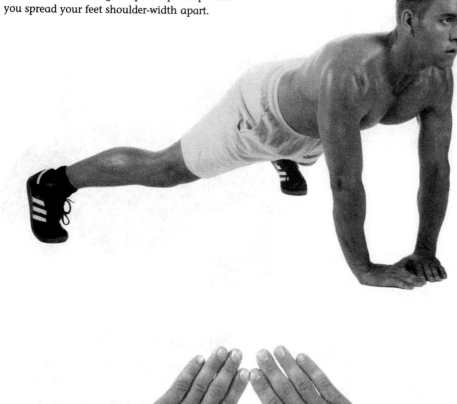

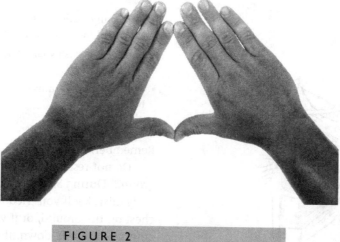

FIGURE 2

Place your hands together, making a diamond shape with your thumbs and index fingers.

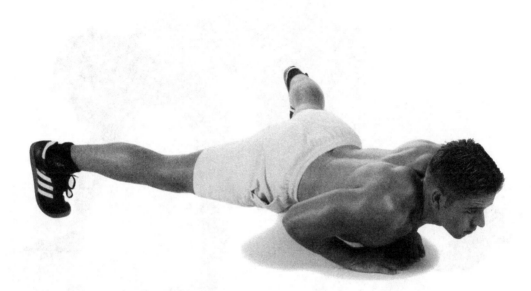

FIGURE 3

- Lower yourself until your chest touches the diamond shape of your hands as shown.

- Raise your body back up to the starting position.

- Reminder: Do not rest your chest on the ground!

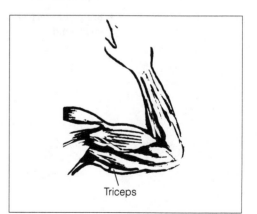

Triceps

27. Dive Bomber

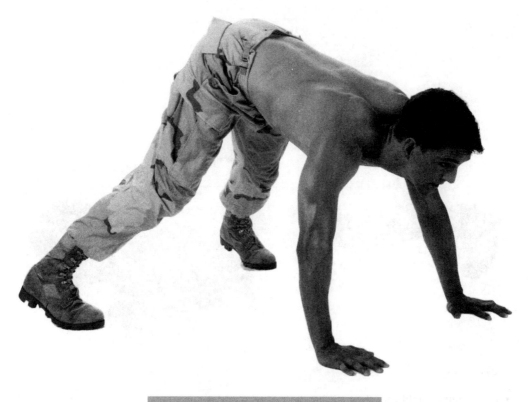

FIGURE 1

- Assume the push-up position. Spread your feet shoulder-width apart, with your buttocks high in the air.
- Bring your feet 12 to 18 inches toward your hands.

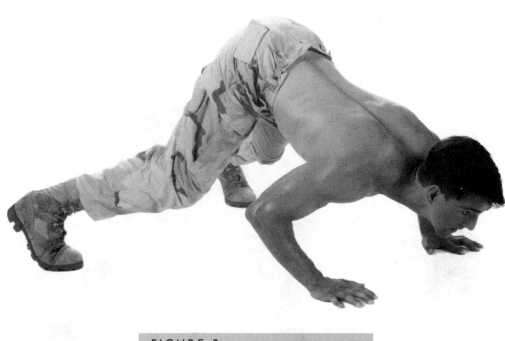

FIGURE 2

Push your head toward the ground.

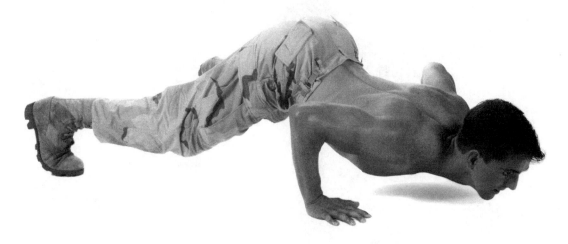

FIGURE 3

- Now pretend you are trying to put your head through a hole at the bottom of a fence.

- Maintain that position for 2 to 3 seconds.

- Using one fluid motion, bring your body back to the original position.

28. Wide-Angle Push-Up

This allows you to work your chest muscles at a different angle, a technique that will help you to increase strength and development.

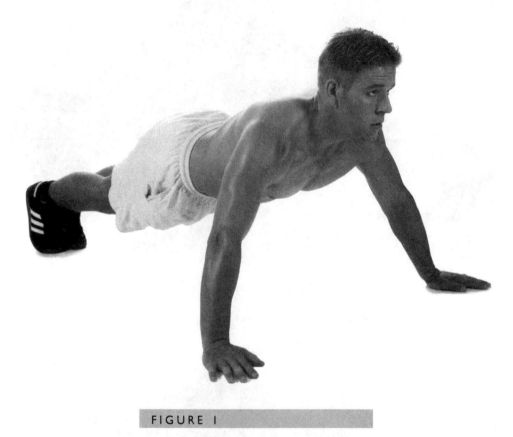

Assume the standard push-up position, but extend your arms farther out, as shown.

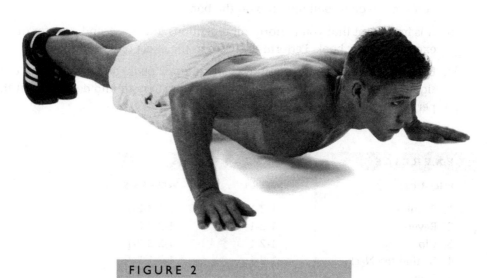

FIGURE 2

Perform the push-up in this position.

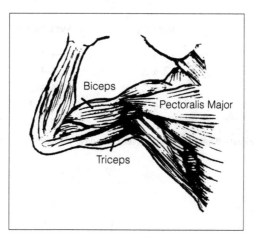

UPPER BODY WORKOUT—BEGINNER

Instructions

1. Find the columns below headed "Exercise" and "Repetition."
2. Under "Exercise" find "Pull-Ups" and go down to "1. Regular."
3. Under "Repetitions," see "Week 1."
4. The repetitions required for this exercise in Week 1 are: "1-2-1."
5. The repetitions are completed as follows:

   Perform 1 regular pull-up; drop off the bar; rest 15 seconds.
   Perform 2 regular pull-ups; drop off the bar; rest 15 seconds.
   Perform 1 regular pull-up; drop off the bar.

6. It is important that you perform all repetitions and 15-second rests for all exercises in this book. Perform exercises in the exact order specified.
7. Exercise repetitions in this format (1 warm-up, 2 peak, and 1 cooldown) are significantly more beneficial to your muscular strength and development than performing other random exercise patterns.

EXERCISE	REPETITIONS		
PULL-UPS	**WEEK 1**	**WEEKS 3–5**	
1. Regular	1-2-1	1-2-3-2-1	
2. Reverse	1-2-1	1-2-3-2-1	
3. Close-Grip	1-2-1	1-2-3-2-1	
4. Behind-the-Neck	1-2-1	1-2-3-2-1	
5. Regular	1-2-1	1-2-3-2-1	
BAR DIPS			
4 sets of 5			
PUSH-UPS	**WEEK 1**	**WEEKS 2–4**	**WEEK 5**
1. Regular	2-4-2	2-4-4-2	2-4-6-4-2
2. Triceps	2-4-2	2-4-4-2	2-4-6-4-2
3. Dive Bomber	2-4-2	2-4-4-2	2-4-6-4-2
4. Wide-Angle	2-4-2	2-4-4-2	2-4-6-4-2

Perform the Upper Body Workout—Beginner program every Monday, Wednesday, and Friday.

UPPER BODY WORKOUT—INTERMEDIATE

Instructions

Complete the Upper Body Workout—Intermediate program as follows:

1. To start, perform this program every Monday, Wednesday, and Friday for four weeks.

2. After four weeks, advance to five times a week (if possible—you will still see benefits even at three times a week).

Perform upper body stretches before and after each workout section.

EXERCISE	REPETITIONS
PULL-UPS	
1. Regular	1-2-3-4-5-4-3-2-1
2. Reverse	1-2-3-4-3-2-1
3. Close-Grip	1-2-3-4-3-2-1
4. Behind-the-Neck	1-2-3-4-3-2-1
5. Commando	1-2-2-1
BAR DIPS	4 sets of 15
PUSH-UPS	
1. Regular	2-4-6-8-10-8-6-4-2
2. Triceps	2-4-6-8-6-4-2
3. Dive Bomber	2-4-6-8-6-4-2
4. Wide-Angle	2-4-6-8-6-4-2

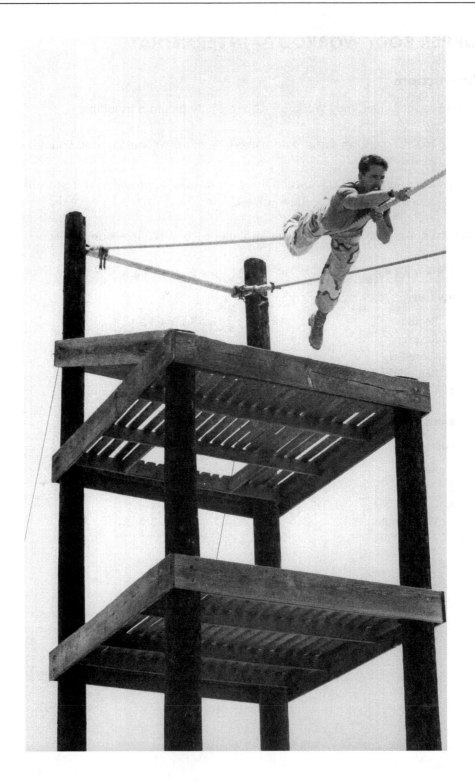

UPPER BODY WORKOUT—ADVANCED

Instructions

Complete the Upper Body Workout—Advanced program five times a week, as follows:

1. To start, perform this program every Monday, Wednesday, and Friday for four weeks.

2. After four weeks, advance to five times a week.

Perform upper body stretches before and after each workout section.

EXERCISE	REPETITIONS
PULL-UPS	
1. Regular	1-2-3-4-5-6-7-8-7-6-5-4-3-2-1
2. Reverse	1-2-3-4-5-6-5-4-3-2-1
3. Close-Grip	1-2-3-4-5-6-5-4-3-2-1
4. Behind-the-Neck	1-2-3-4-5-6-5-4-3-2-1
5. Commando	1-2-3-4-3-2-1
BAR DIPS	4 sets of 20
PUSH-UPS	
1. Regular	2-4-6-8-10-12-14-12-10-8-6-4-2
2. Triceps	2-4-6-8-10-12-10-8-6-4-2
3. Dive Bomber	2-4-6-8-10-12-10-8-6-4-2
4. Wide-Angle	2-4-6-8-10-12-10-8-6-4-2

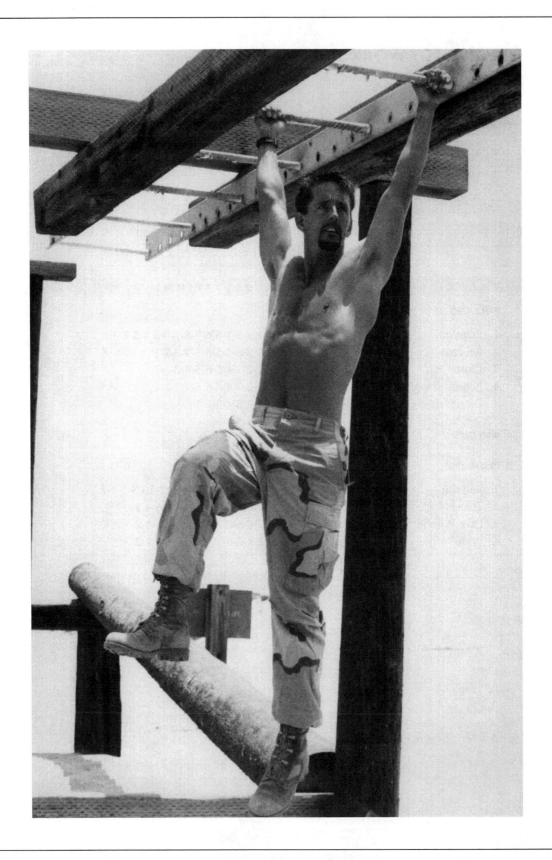

3. Lower Body Workout

During SEAL training I had to do thousands and thousands of sit-ups although they are no longer part of the SEAL workout. Without proper form, I would not have been able to keep up or maintain a healthy back.

Pay strict attention to these instructions and use the pictures to help you learn proper form. Doing these exercises *as instructed* will get your abs into phenomenal condition; it will also keep you from injuring yourself.

In-between Lower Body Workout exercises, it is wise to use the cobra stretch (page 34) to loosen up your abdominals. Perform this stretch every third exercise.

At the end of each week increase your repetitions by increments of five. If one week is not enough time to reach your goals, then increase every two weeks. Keep increasing until you reach 60. When you are comfortable with 60 and ready to go on to 65—*stop!*

Now you are ready to move on to the advanced stage.

This is the same as the beginning of the intermediate stage, except you perform two sets of 35 repetitions each—instead of one set of 60. Once again, continue to increase by increments of five until you reach 60 per set. At this point, increase to three sets.

Never be satisfied with the fitness level you are working on, until you reach your final goal. Continually push yourself to go past your limits. Only when you push yourself will you be capable of achieving the results and fitness level you desire.

Let's get started!

TRAINING TIP

Proper Hand Position and General Rules for Abdominal Exercises

To avoid injuries while doing abdominal exercises, remember these points:

1. Do not place your hands behind your neck, because this causes too much strain on your neck, upper and lower back, and legs.

2. Avoid bringing your chest up to your thighs. This also puts too much strain on your back.

3. Do not rock during your abdominal exercises.

4. Perform each abdominal exercise with strict movements to isolate your abdominals.

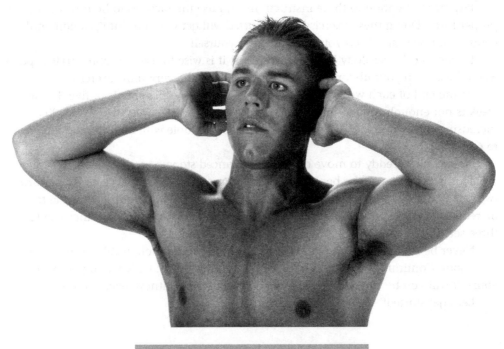

FIGURE 1

- Fingers should be gently touching the outer parts of the ears.

- *Do not* place your hands behind your neck, as this can cause injury to the neck.

29. Half Sit-Up

While doing half sit-ups, be sure to lower your upper body *slowly* to avoid injuring your back.

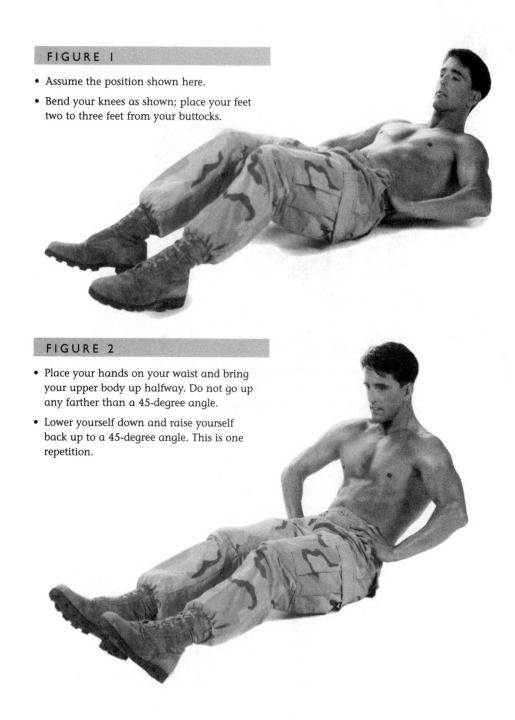

FIGURE 1

- Assume the position shown here.
- Bend your knees as shown; place your feet two to three feet from your buttocks.

FIGURE 2

- Place your hands on your waist and bring your upper body up halfway. Do not go up any farther than a 45-degree angle.
- Lower yourself down and raise yourself back up to a 45-degree angle. This is one repetition.

30. Hand-to-Toe

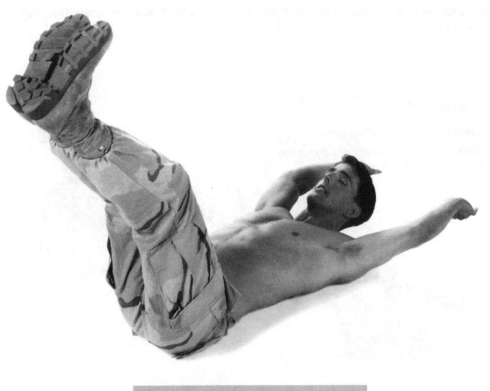

FIGURE 1

- Lie down on your back with your arms over your head.
- Raise your legs at a 90-degree angle.

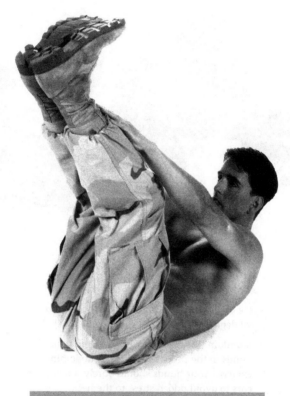

FIGURE 2

- Raise your upper body and try to touch your toes. It is OK if you cannot touch your toes. Just go for your ankles or knees. As your physical fitness and flexibility improve, go for your toes.

- Keep your legs as straight as possible throughout the entire motion; your legs will bend slightly naturally.

- It is extremely important to raise your shoulder blades off the ground, or you will defeat the purpose of this exercise.

31. Crunch

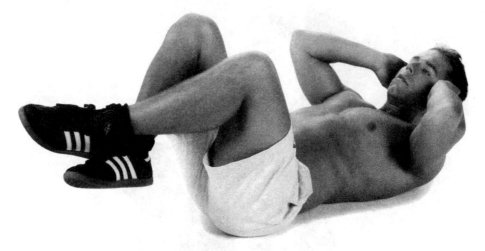

FIGURE 1

- Lie on your back and raise your knees at a 90-degree angle.

- Maintain this position while placing your hands in the proper position for abdominal exercise. Your hands should barely touch your ears to avoid added stress to the neck.

- Do not allow your shoulders to touch the ground.

- Isolate your stomach muscles by keeping them tight during the entire movement.

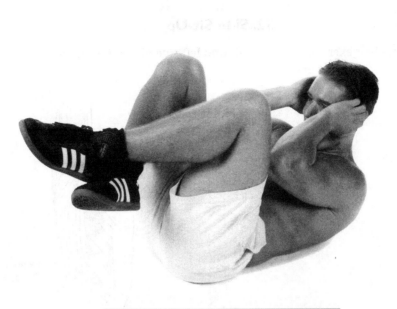

FIGURE 2

- Raise your upper body toward your thighs, so your elbows touch them; use your abdominal muscles to pull you up.

- Once you have reached your thighs, lower yourself back down with control.

32. Side Sit-Up

This is an excellent exercise for the right- and left-side abdominal muscles.

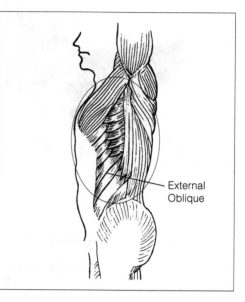

External
Oblique

FIGURE I

- Lie down in the sit-up position and place your right ankle on your left knee, so that your right knee is perpendicular to your body.

- Place your hands in the standard position, applying little or no pressure on your ears.

- Do not allow your shoulders to touch the ground.

- Maintain maximum stomach-muscle tightness during this entire movement.

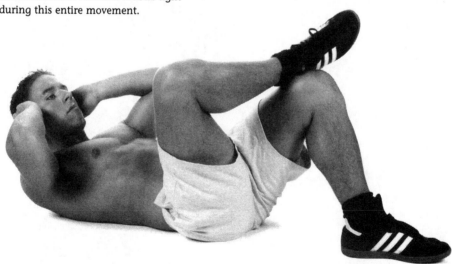

FIGURE 2

Raise your upper body so that your left elbow touches your right knee, and then slowly bring yourself back down.

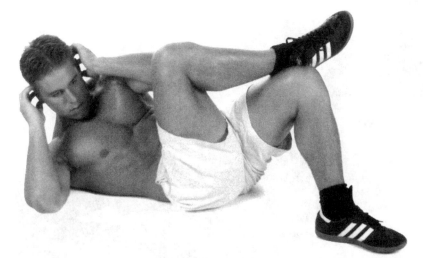

FIGURE 3

Once you have finished with the left side, switch legs and work your right side.

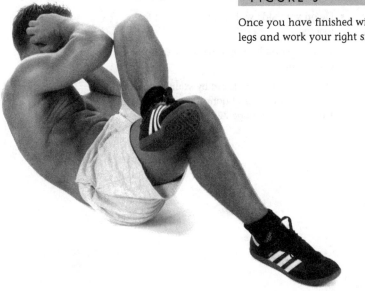

33. Oblique

To get the full effect of this exercise, technique is extremely important.

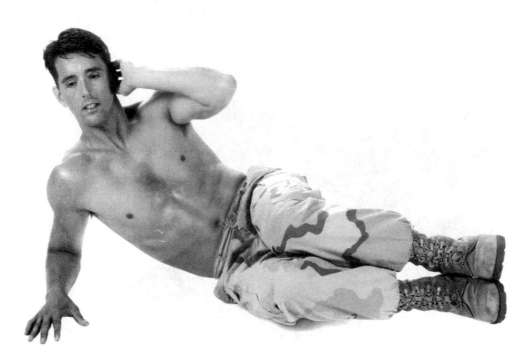

FIGURE 1

- Lie on your side with your knees and feet together.
- Your upper body should be propped up on your elbow.
- Place your opposite hand by your ear, in the correct manner for abdominal exercises (see Training Tip on page 72).

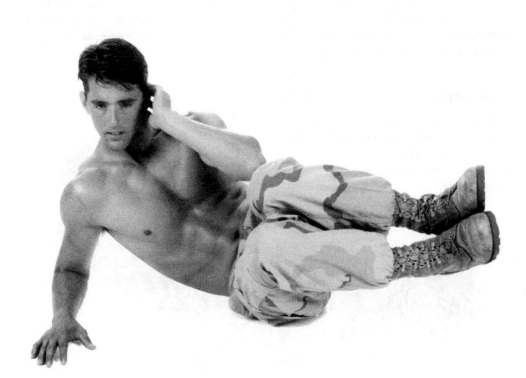

FIGURE 2

- Here is the key part! Raise your feet straight up, as if someone has tied a string to your feet and is pulling it.

- Curl your upper body until your elbow is touching your knees. Do not make the mistake of bringing your knees to your chest. Remember that the legs are raised; then you curl your upper body into them.

- Once you have completed the recommended repetitions, switch sides and begin the process over again.

34. Flutter Kick

Do not be concerned about speed in this exercise. This is a technique exercise. This exercise is to be done on a four count. As you raise each foot up to the 36-inch mark, start counting. On the fourth count, say the cumulative total. For example: 1-2-3-**1**, 1-2-3-**2**, 1-2-3-**3**, 1-2-3-**4**, and so on.

FIGURE 1

- Lie on your back and place your hands palms-down under your buttocks. This will give your hips support.
- Raise both your feet six inches. Keep your legs straight.

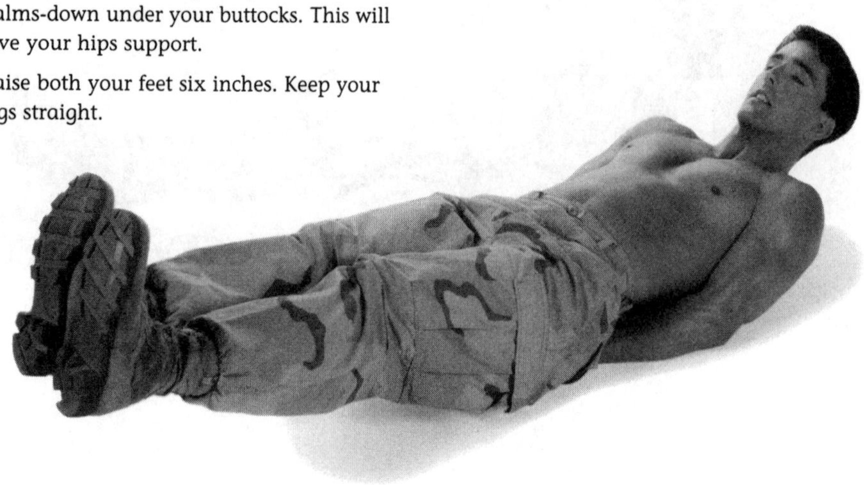

FIGURE 2

Raise your right foot until it is approximately 36 inches off the ground, then lower it back down to the starting position.

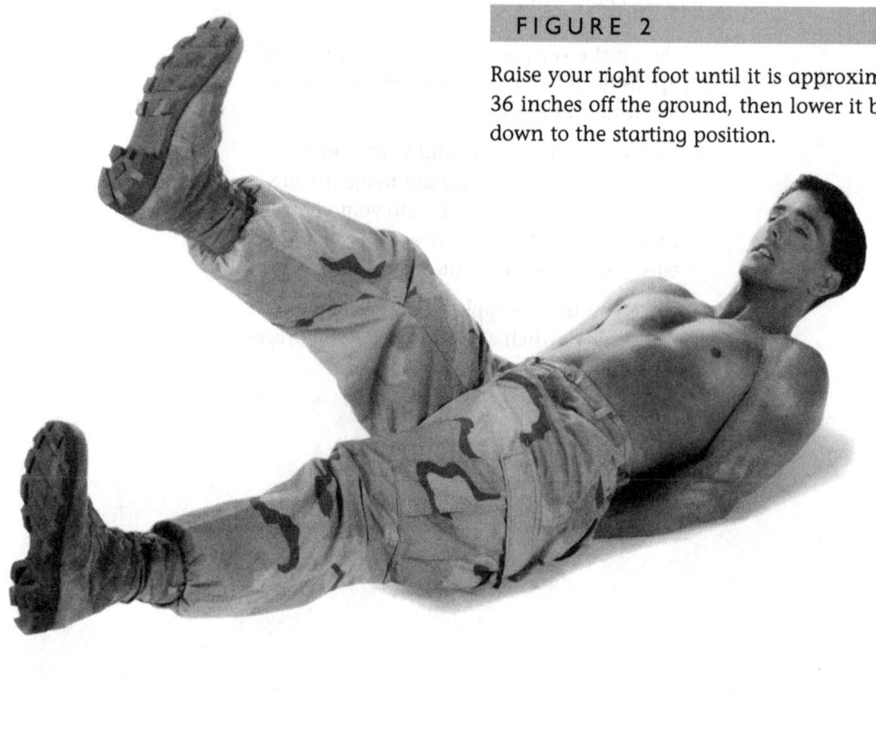

FIGURE 3

As you do so, raise your left foot 36 inches off the ground.

FIGURE 4

- Bring your left foot back down and raise your right foot back up to the 36-inch mark.
- Continue alternating in a fluid motion.

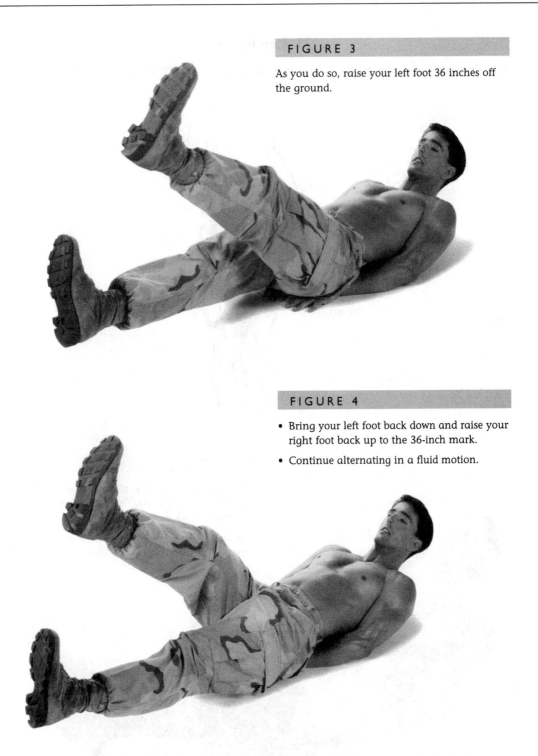

In the advanced section, when doing higher reps, it is recommended that you do this exercise three times a week or every other day.

35. Leg Raise

Remember to isolate your abdominal muscles when performing this exercise.

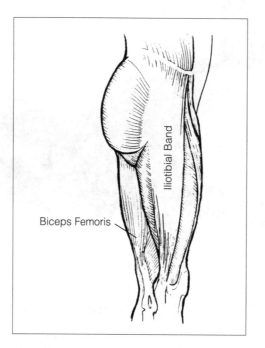

Iliotibial Band

Biceps Femoris

FIGURE I

- Lie down on your back, placing your hands palms-down under your buttocks. This will give your back support.

- Raise your feet six inches off the ground; keep your heels together.

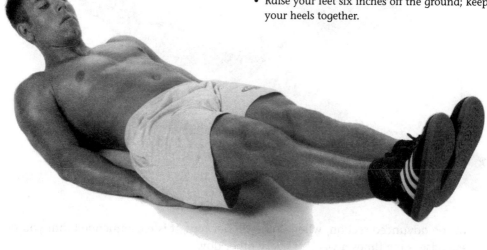

FIGURE 2

Raise your legs up to 36 inches, heels together, as shown.

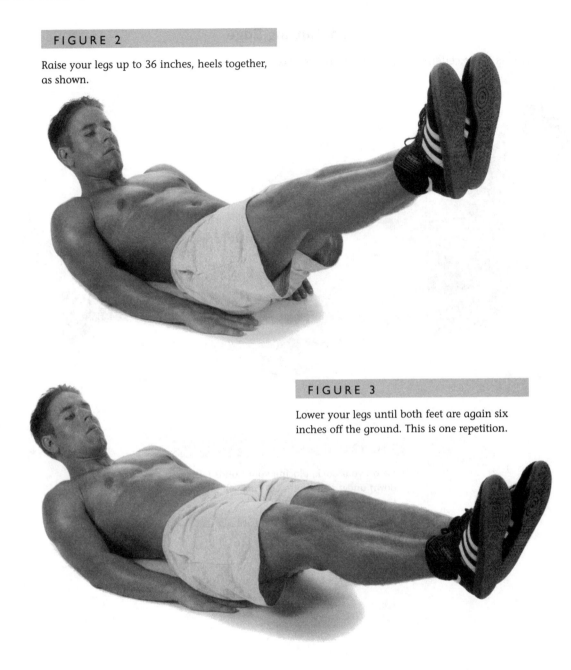

FIGURE 3

Lower your legs until both feet are again six inches off the ground. This is one repetition.

If you are new to exercising, or if it has been a while, it is recommended that this exercise be done with one leg on the ground to relieve tension on the lower back. Once you finish one repetition, switch legs.

36. Cutting Edge

This is an excellent lower-abdominal exercise.

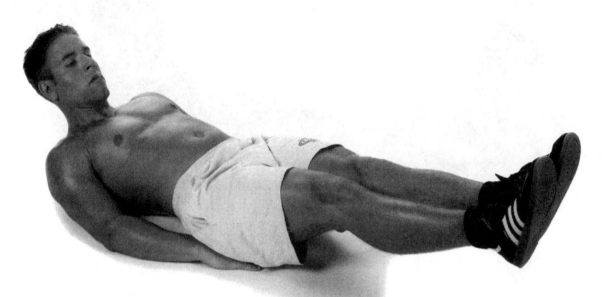

FIGURE 1

- Lie on your back, placing your hands palms-down under your buttocks. This will give your back support.

- Raise your legs, heels together, about six inches off the ground.

FIGURE 2

- Spread your legs apart 48 inches, or just past shoulder width, and bring them back together. This is one repetition.

- Continue in this manner until you have completed the required number of repetitions.

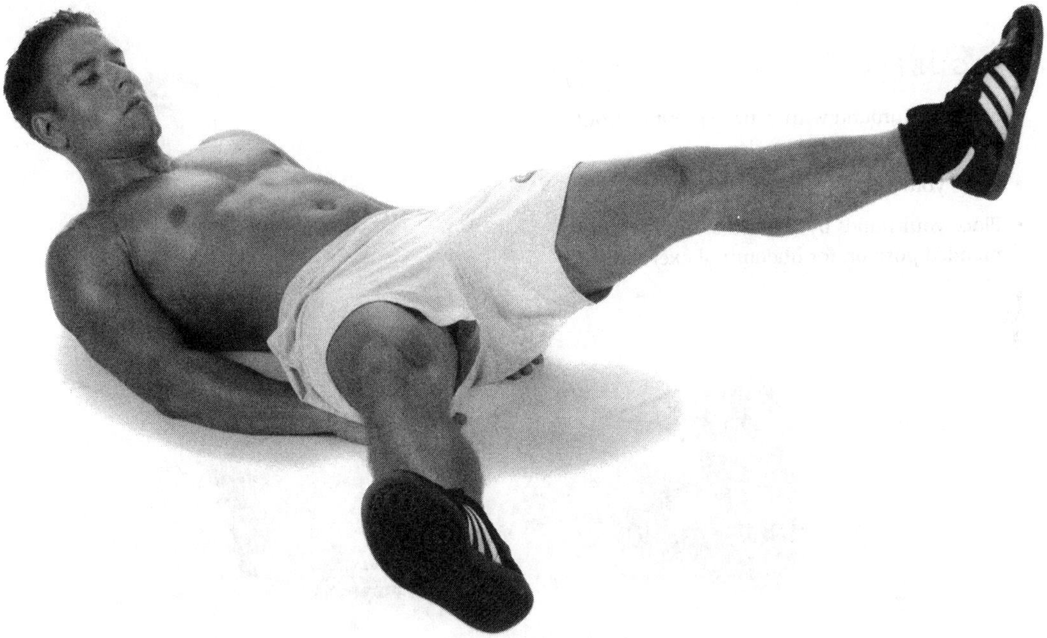

FIGURE 3

Then bring your feet together again, one last time, and lower both feet to the ground.

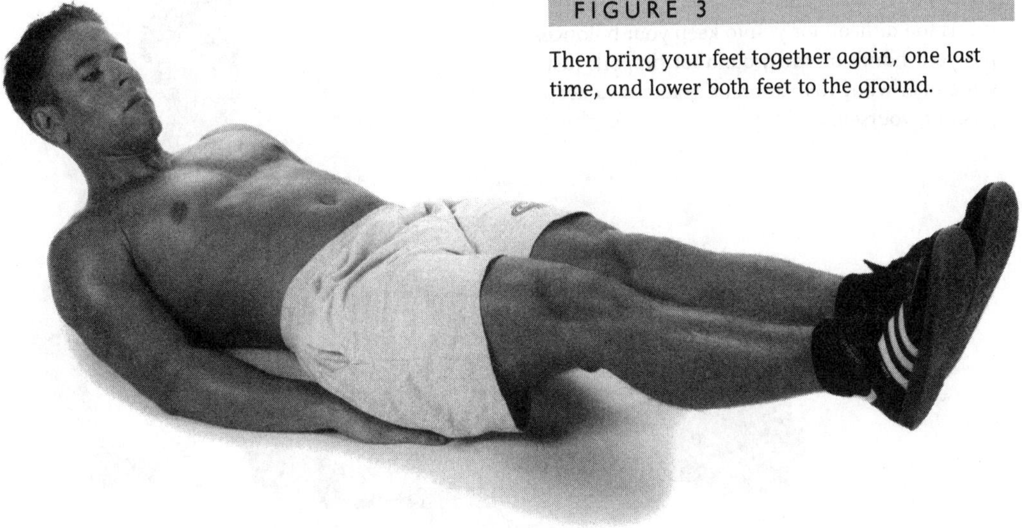

37. Knee Bend

There is a trick to performing this exercise that will allow you to keep your balance more easily. Extend your legs out straight, heels on the ground. Begin leaning back, keeping your hands in their proper position by your ears. The moment your feet begin to rise off the ground, you've found your equilibrium point. This is the best position in which to perform this exercise.

FIGURE 1

- Sit on the ground with your legs out in front of you at a 45-degree angle.

- Raise your feet six inches.

- Place your hands by your ears, in the recommended position for abdominal exercise.

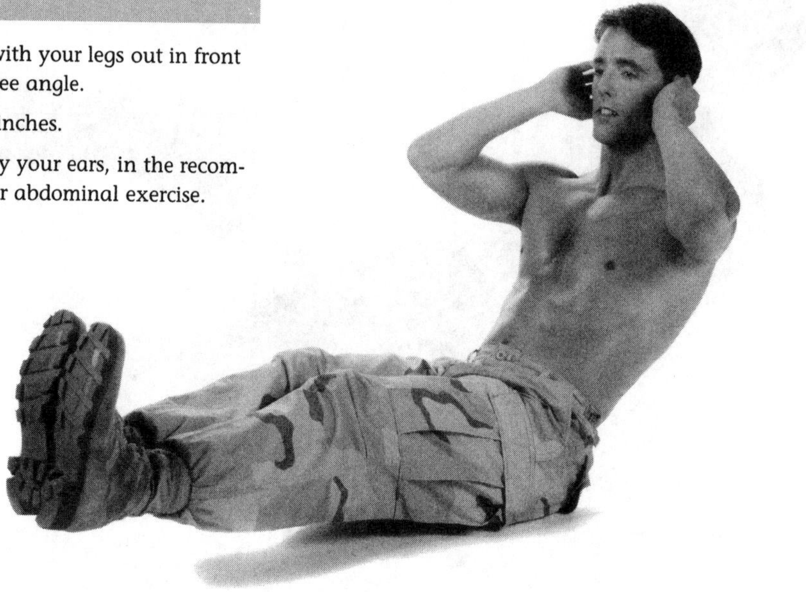

FIGURE 2

If it is too difficult for you to keep your balance, put your hands on the ground for support. Just remember what your ultimate goal is and keep pushing yourself.

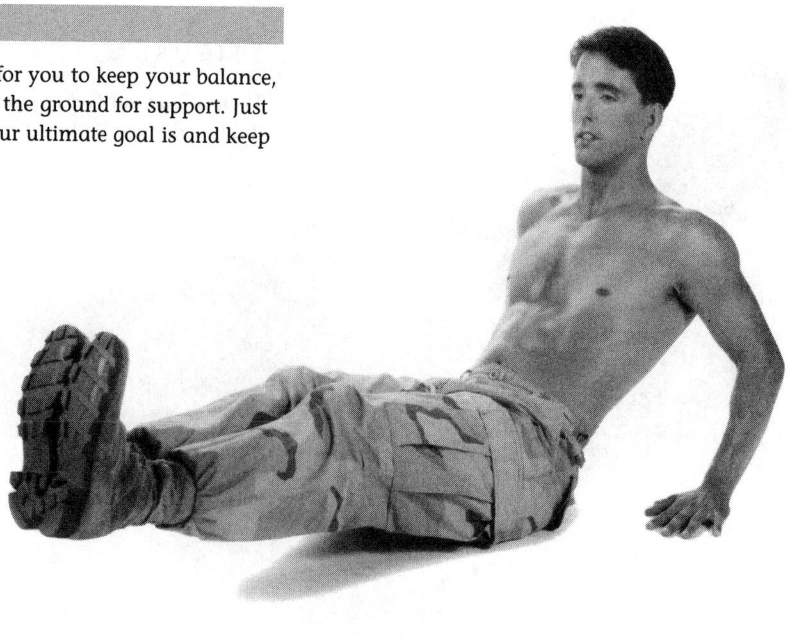

FIGURE 3

- Bring your knees toward your chest in a smooth, fluid motion.
- Do not allow your feet to touch the ground!

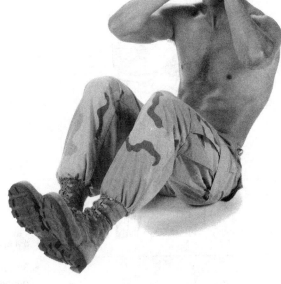

FIGURE 4

Extend your legs back out again until they are straight.

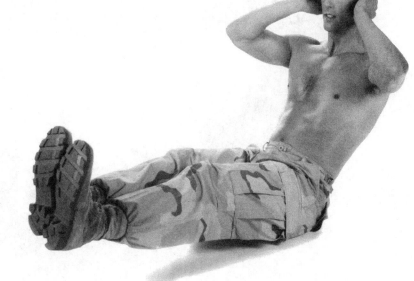

38. Abdominal Twister

This exercise requires a lot of balance and control with your abdominal muscles. Only with time and practice will this exercise become more efficient and smooth.

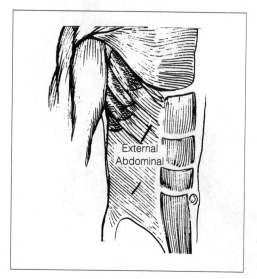

External
Abdominal

FIGURE 1

- Sit on the ground with your back at a 45-degree angle.
- Raise your legs three inches off the ground.

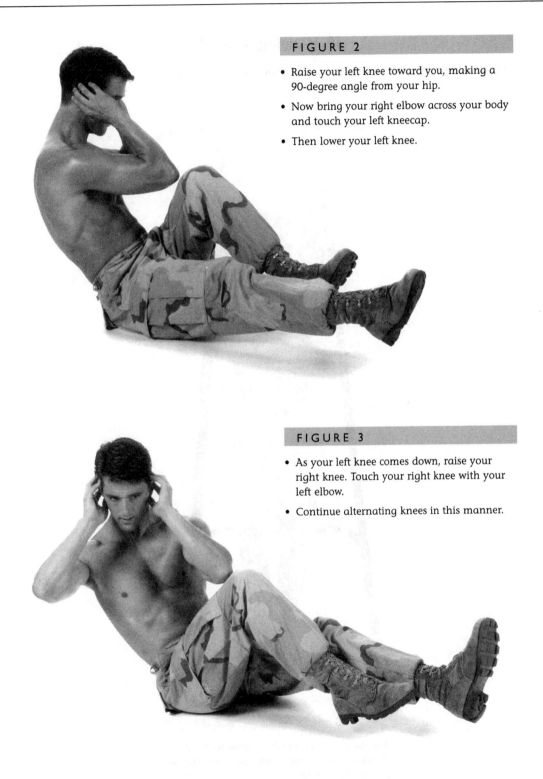

FIGURE 2

- Raise your left knee toward you, making a 90-degree angle from your hip.
- Now bring your right elbow across your body and touch your left kneecap.
- Then lower your left knee.

FIGURE 3

- As your left knee comes down, raise your right knee. Touch your right knee with your left elbow.
- Continue alternating knees in this manner.

39. Hanging Knee-Up

You must have access to a secure pull-up bar to perform this exercise.

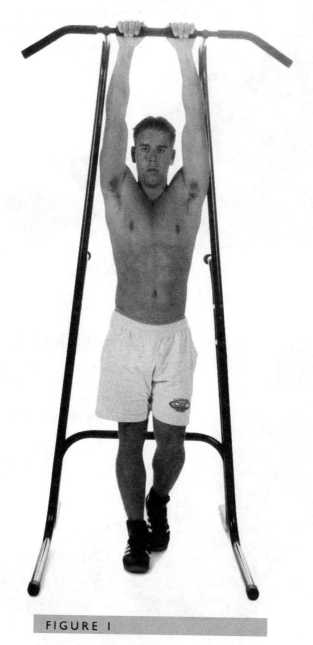

FIGURE I

Assume the starting position shown above. The object is to keep your upper body stable while performing this exercise.

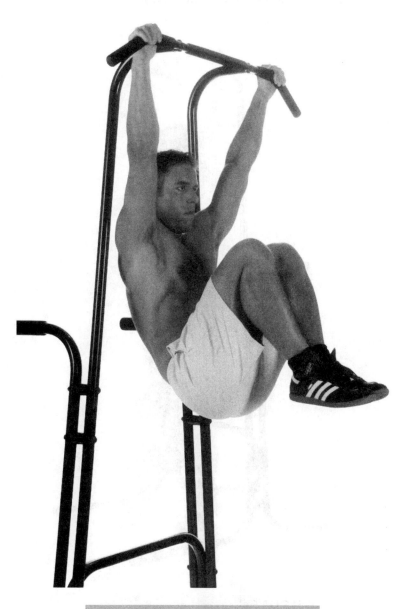

FIGURE 2

- Raise your knees up to your chest, so that your thighs are flush against your stomach.

- Slowly lower your knees until your legs are straight. To avoid putting too much strain on your back, do not drop your legs down quickly.

40. Hanging Leg-Up

To do this exercise you must have access to a secure pull-up bar. This is a very difficult exercise, so just take your time and do the best you can.

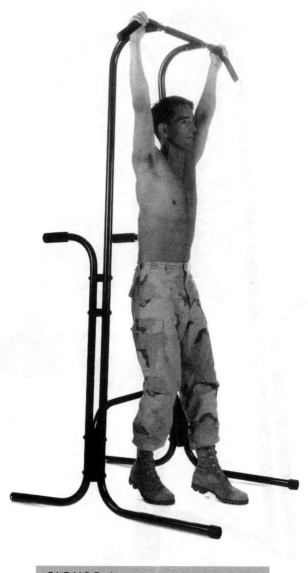

FIGURE 1

Hang from your pull-up bar with a firm grip. Your hands should grasp the bar at slightly beyond shoulder width.

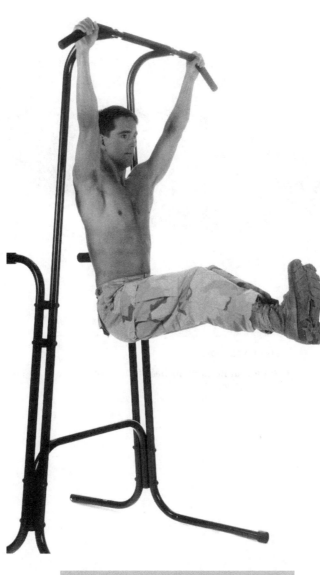

FIGURE 2

- Raise your feet up toward your head, as high as you can, while keeping your upper body as stable as possible.

- To avoid back injury, lower your legs slowly.

- Do not rock. Instead isolate your abs and allow them to pull your legs up.

41. Floor Knee-Up

If you can't do the hanging leg-up because you do not have access to a pull-up bar, you can get the same effect with this exercise.

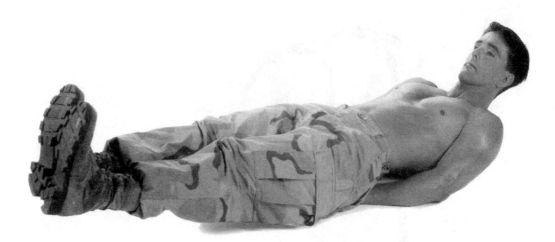

FIGURE 1

- Lie on your back.
- Raise your heels six inches off the ground.

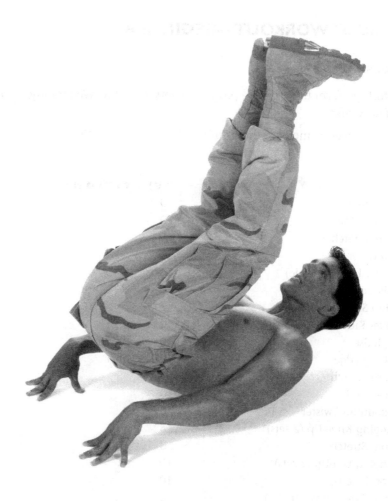

FIGURE 2

- Now bring your knees toward your chest, as shown above.

- To prevent injury, when curling your legs to your chest do not let your lower back move more than 90° from your starting prone position.

- The key to this exercise is that when you lower your legs you do not let your feet touch the ground.

- Only when the set is over may you lower your feet to the ground. *No cheating!*

LOWER BODY WORKOUT—BEGINNER

Instructions

1. To start, perform this exercise program every Monday, Wednesday, and Friday for four weeks.

2. After four weeks, increase the number of repetitions by five.

EXERCISE	REPETITIONS
1. Half Sit-Up	10
2. Hand-to-Toe	10
3. Cobra Stretch	3
4. Crunch	10
5. Side Sit-Up (each side)	10
6. Oblique (each side)	10
7. Cobra Stretch	3
8. Flutter Kick	10 (4 count)
9. Leg Raise	10
10. Cutting Edge	10 (4 count)
11. Cobra Stretch	3
12. Knee Bend	10
13. Abdominal Twister	10
14. Hanging Knee-Up (2 sets)*	5
15. Cobra Stretch	3
16. Hanging Leg-Up (2 sets)*	10
17. Floor Knee-Up	10
18. Trunk Extensions (stretch)	5

* Optional

LOWER BODY WORKOUT—INTERMEDIATE

Instructions

1. To start, perform this exercise program every Monday, Wednesday, and Friday for four weeks.

2. After four weeks, advance your routine by five reps.

EXERCISE	REPETITIONS
1. Half Sit-Up	30
2. Hand-to-Toe	30
3. Cobra Stretch	3
4. Crunch	30
5. Side Sit-Up (each side)	30
6. Oblique (each side)	30
7. Cobra Stretch	3
8. Flutter Kick	20 (4 count)
9. Leg Raise	30
10. Cutting Edge	20 (4 count)
11. Cobra Stretch	3
12. Knee Bend	30
13. Abdominal Twister	30
14. Hanging Knee-Up (2 sets)*	15
15. Cobra Stretch	3
16. Hanging Leg-Up (2 sets)*	15
17. Floor Knee-Up	30
18. Trunk Extensions (stretch)	5

* Optional

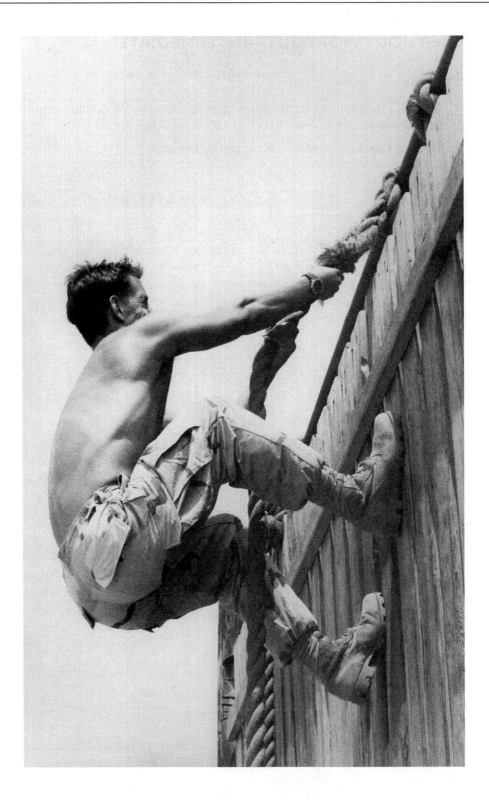

LOWER BODY WORKOUT—ADVANCED

Instructions

1. You will now be doing two sets of each exercise.

2. Complete a full cycle (one set) before moving on to the second cycle.

3. Perform the following exercise program five times a week.

EXERCISE	REPETITION
1. Half Sit-Up	2 × 35
2. Hand-to-Toe	2 × 35
3. Cobra Stretch	3
4. Crunch	2 × 35
5. Side Sit-Up (each side)	2 × 35
6. Oblique (each side)	2 × 35
7. Cobra Stretch	3
8. Flutter Kick	2 × 30 (4 count)
9. Leg Raise	2 × 35
10. Cutting Edge	2 × 30 (4 count)
11. Cobra Stretch	3
12. Knee Bend	2 × 35
13. Abdominal Twister	2 × 35
14. Hanging Knee-Up	2 × 35
15. Cobra Stretch	3
16. Hanging Leg-Up	2 × 35
17. Floor Knee-Up	2 × 35
18. Trunk Extensions (stretch)	10

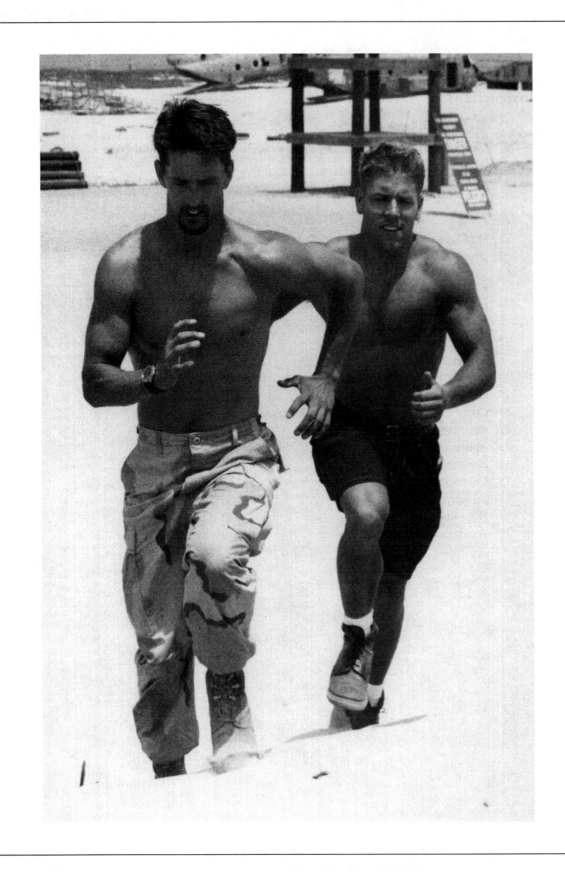

4. Running

Running can be a controversial subject. Some swear by running; others have nothing good to say about it. I do not have a Ph.D. in physiology or science, but running has been a major part of my life and career, and I can attest to the fact that you can receive great joy from it, not only because of the physical benefits but also because of the peace of mind that you can get from it.

For SEALs at BUD/S, running is practically a daily ritual. Men have been made and men have been broken by excruciating runs during SEAL training. Each SEAL team runs three times a week, and almost everyone runs on their own during the other days of the week. Of course, when you are training for an op (operation/mission) you usually do not have time to yourself. As a Navy SEAL, I have fond memories and also bitter memories of running during my training at BUD/S.

I've always enjoyed heading out to an empty, tourist-free beach and running as the sun sets. I pick a nice, steady pace, and as the sun goes down I feel my worries and concerns leaving along with it. There is nothing quite like it. What a great way to get away from it all and relieve some tension.

Then there are the bitter memories of running during SEAL training. Our physical training leader, Instructor Jared, had just finished exercising us to death and was standing up front, ready to take us out for a run. After a grueling session, this guy hadn't even broken a sweat!

Whenever Instructor Jared ran us, we knew it was going to be a death march. He may not have been the fastest instructor at BUD/S, but his stamina was unbelievable. I would rather run behind the fastest instructor on a long road run, than have to run behind an instructor who runs up and down sand berms and through soft sand. Sure enough—that's where Instructor Jared took us. He never broke stride—not even in the softest sands!

Instructor Jared also usually had the biggest goon squad. The goon squad is the unfortunate group of runners who fall behind the leader, usually lagging about 30 to 60 yards back (varying on each instructor's current mood). Instructor Jared would put us through grueling runs, hoping to create a big goon squad. The goon squad is given a warning to catch up—or else. If they don't catch up, they get hammered with more and more intensive exercise. It is not uncommon to see someone pass out or drop from fatigue, just trying to keep up with the team. This is where I learned to dig deep down inside myself to accomplish things I'd never known I was capable of doing.

If you have never included running in your training program, or if you have not been running in a long time, I recommend starting out very slowly to prevent shin splints and stress fractures. I also recommend running at the end of your workout, since your muscles will be good and warm, even if they are a little tired from exercising. This is the best time for growth—and you will not have to run a long distance to get the same effect.

Try to add variety to your running, to spice it up a little. Like anything done over and over again, running can become very boring if you always do it on the same course and in the same manner. I recommend running long distances on Mondays, Wednesdays, and Fridays. On Tuesdays and Thursdays, go to a nearby track and do wind sprints.[1] Another great way to work on speed, strength, and stamina is by doing sprints *uphill*. This is an awesome workout! I know because I had to do hundreds of sprints up soft sand dunes during BUD/S training. The goal is to work on both speed and endurance. By following this program, you will achieve both.

I realize that most people dislike sprints, but by ordering this workout program you have proven that you are not just *anyone*. You are someone who's ready to push yourself to the limit to achieve a rock-hard body.

By doing sprints you train the muscle fibers in your legs to react quickly. This will generate greater development and improve your body's speed in short-burst situations. Your legs are made up of fast twitch fibers and slow twitch fibers. By running long distances, you work the slow twitch fibers. Include wind sprints once a week to work the fast twitch fibers. Sprints will improve the overall development of your legs.

Be creative and make running enjoyable. Once your running or sprint session is finished, spend a little time stretching out. I'm not talking about a marathon stretch session—just a couple of minutes of stretching will help you prevent injuries and improve flexibility.

---

[1] A "wind sprint" is short-distance running, going back and forth from one designated spot to another, an all-out burst of running as fast as you can.

Running Workout—Beginner

First Week

Monday	1 mile
Tuesday	$1/2$-mile interval or 900 yards: jogging first 200 yards, then sprinting for 100 yards, and so on, up to 900 yards
Wednesday	1 mile
Thursday	Sprint 100 yards and jog 100 yards, up to 900 yards
Friday	1 mile

Second Week

Monday	1 mile
Tuesday	Stair sprints (stairs, bleachers, hills), 5 minutes total time[1]
Wednesday	1 mile
Thursday	$1/2$-mile interval or 900 yards (see above explanation)
Friday	$1^1/2$ miles

[1] Pick a 25-foot section of stairs to sprint up—then jog down. You want to continue to push yourself. No walking in this exercise! Each person's fitness level varies, so take it slow to find your limitation. If you have never sprinted up stairs before, you'll find out that it is tougher than it looks. Do not attempt the Advanced level straight out of the gate. Your stamina will increase, but you must work toward it with moderation. Increase your distance $1/2$ mile every two weeks.

Running Workout—Intermediate

First Week

Monday	3 miles
Tuesday	1-mile interval or 1,800 yards: jogging first 300 yards, sprinting for 150 yards, jogging 300 yards, and so on, up to 1,800 yards
Wednesday	3 miles
Thursday	Jog 300 yards, sprint 150 yards, and so on, up to 1,800 yards
Friday	3 miles

Second Week

Monday	3 miles
Tuesday	Stair sprints, 10 minutes total time (50 feet maximum height)
Wednesday	3 miles
Thursday	1-mile interval or 1,800 yards (see above explanation)
Friday	3^1/2 miles

Running Workout—Advanced

First Week

Monday	4 miles
Tuesday	1½-mile interval, or 2,700 yards: jogging 300 yards, sprinting 150 yards, jogging 300 yards, and so on, up to 2,700 yards
Wednesday	4 miles
Thursday	Jog 300 yards, sprint 150 yards, up to 2,700 yards
Friday	4 miles

Second Week

Monday	4 miles
Tuesday	Stair sprints, 15 minutes total (100 feet maximum height)
Wednesday	4 miles
Thursday	1½-mile interval: jogging 300 yards, sprinting 150 yards, jogging 300 yards, and so on, up to 2,700 yards
Friday	4½ miles

Once you have reached the advanced program, your progress does not stop. This program is just the minimum, which means you will continue to increase in increments of a half-mile every two weeks, up to six miles. You can stay at this level or continue on.

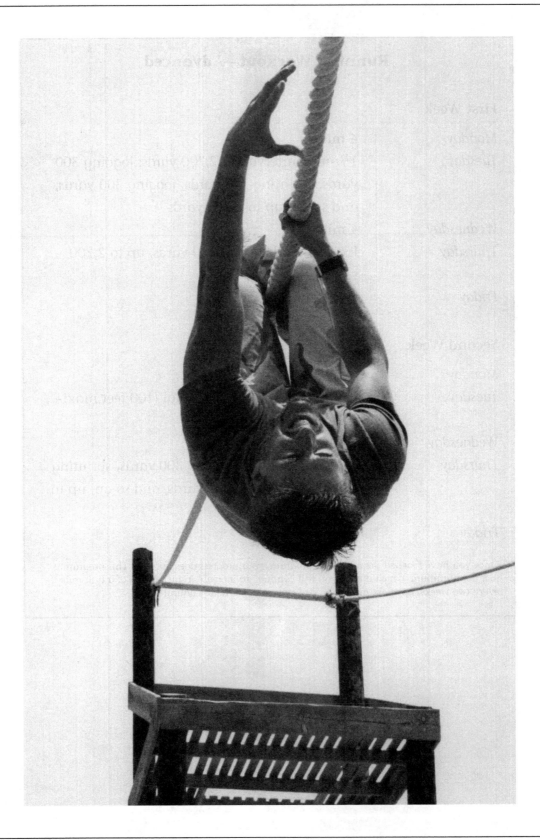

5. Swimming

Many people admire the sleek and hard muscles of swimmers. It seems as though swimmers have every muscle developed, with no weak areas. Men and women dream of being as toned as swimmers. The thing to remember is that all these aspirations and dreams will remain just that—if you don't jump in and get wet.

Unfortunately, not everyone has access to a swimming pool. If you don't, just remember the things I'm going to discuss and when you do have access to a pool, use them then. You don't have to have a swimming pool in your backyard. There are pools at health clubs, community centers, high schools, and colleges. Wherever the most convenient pool may be, try to find regular access to it because swimming is probably the best way to improve your overall fitness.

If swimming is new to you, take lessons from a certified instructor. If you wanted to skydive, you wouldn't grab a parachute and jump—you would take lessons from a qualified instructor who takes the time to demonstrate proper technique, proper gear, and so on. Same with swimming. To avoid drowning you must learn proper technique, and an instructor also will prevent you from picking up any bad habits. Take this recommendation and your training regimen will be much more enjoyable.

Swimming should be broken up into several strokes. During BUD/S training we were taught two strokes: freestyle and the side stroke [or UDT stroke]. We achieved the best results when we alternated between using fins and going barefoot.

I recommend using swimming fins to assist your strokes, and goggles to protect your eyes from chlorine. These products are available at your local sporting goods store. Another useful item for swimming is a flotation device that allows you to run in the pool. This will allow you to jog in the pool with zero stress on the joints.

Swimming can be one of the most beneficial forms of exercise you'll ever do. Once again, before you begin any strenuous exercise, remember to stretch. The upper body stretches will work great for your swimming routine (see pages 4–17).

SEALs are like fish in the water; we are extremely comfortable there. During BUD/S training we swam up to 5,000 yards a day.

It was amazing to see the great shape that swimming helped us to achieve. You can achieve the same extraordinary results. So jump in!

Swimming Workout—Beginner

Monday	Freestyle for 600 yards
Tuesday	Breast stroke for 300 yards
Wednesday	Freestyle for 600 yards
Thursday	Side stroke for 600 yards
Friday	Freestyle for 600 yards

Every two weeks increase your distance 100 yards.

Swimming Workout—Intermediate

Monday	Freestyle for 1,200 yards
Tuesday	Breast stroke for 600 yards
Wednesday	Freestyle for 1,200 yards
Thursday	Side stroke for 1,200 yards
Friday	Freestyle stroke for 1,200 yards

Every two weeks increase your distance 100 yards.

SWIMMING

Swimming Workout—Advanced

Monday	Freestyle for 1,800 yards
Tuesday	Breast stroke for 900 yards
Wednesday	Freestyle for 1,800 yards
Thursday	Side stroke for 1,800 yards
Friday	Freestyle for 1,800 yards

Every two weeks increase your distance 100 yards.

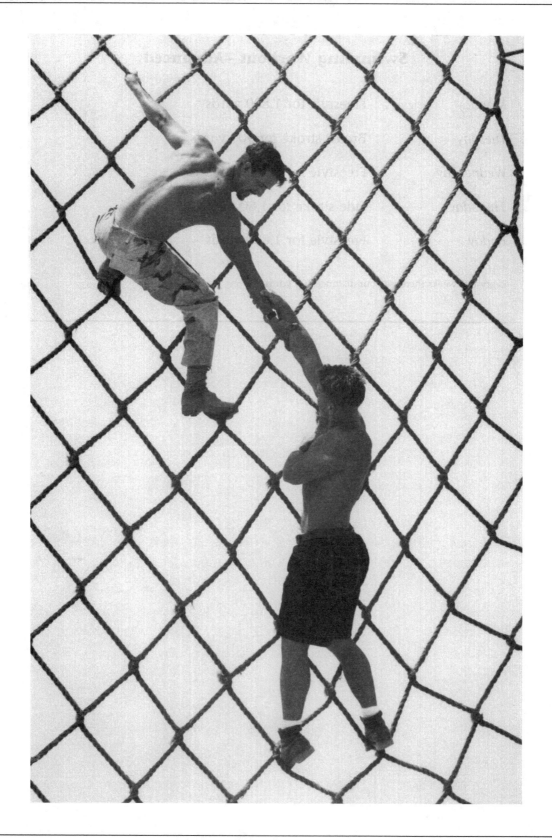

6. Combined Program

Combined Program—Beginner

First Week

Monday	1-mile run
Tuesday	Freestyle stroke for 600 yards
Wednesday	900-yard interval: jog 300 yards, sprint 150 yards, jog 300 yards, and so on, up to 900 yards
Thursday	Freestyle stroke for 400 yards, breast stroke for 200 yards
Friday	1-mile run

Second Week

Monday	1-mile run
Tuesday	Freestyle stroke for 600 yards
Wednesday	Stair sprints, 25 feet, 5 minutes
Thursday	Freestyle stroke for 400 yards, side stroke for 200 yards
Friday	$1^1/_2$-mile run

Combined Program—Intermediate

First Week

Monday	3-mile run
Tuesday	Freestyle stroke for 1,200 yards
Wednesday	1,800-yard interval: jog 300 yards, sprint 150 yards, jog 300 yards, and so on, up to 1,800 yards
Thursday	Freestyle for 1,200 yards
Friday	3-mile run

Second Week

Monday	3-mile run
Tuesday	Freestyle stroke for 1,200 yards
Wednesday	Stair sprints, 50 feet, 10 minutes
Thursday	Freestyle stroke for 800 yards, side stroke for 400 yards
Friday	3$^{1}/_{2}$-mile run

Combined Program—Advanced

First Week

Monday	4-mile run
Tuesday	Freestyle stroke for 1,800 yards
Wednesday	$1^1/_2$-mile interval: jog 300 yards, sprint 150 yards, jog 300 yards, and so on, up to 2,700 yards
Thursday	Freestyle for 1,200 yards, breast stroke for 600 yards
Friday	4-mile run

Second Week

Monday	4-mile run
Tuesday	Freestyle for 1,800 yards
Wednesday	Stair sprint, 100 feet, 15 minutes
Thursday	Freestyle stroke for 1,200 yards, side stroke for 600 yards
Friday	$4^1/_2$-mile run

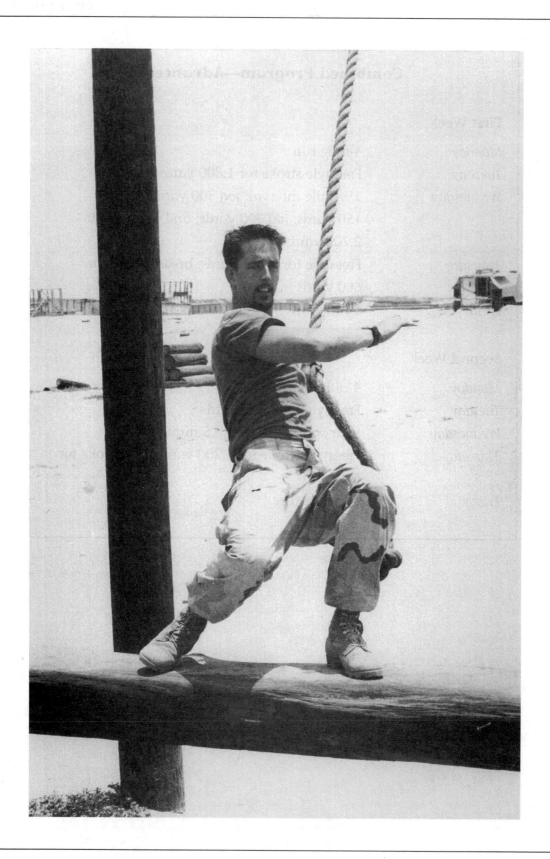

7. Cooldown

Cooling down is an important step in the recovery of your muscles. Any time you engage in strenuous exercise it is necessary to stretch out your muscles to prevent pulls and intense soreness. You are not going to avoid soreness—you are going to be sore for about the first two weeks. But don't worry, your body will adjust to your new routine. Soreness means growth or, as we say in training, "Soreness is weakness leaving the body." There is a difference between soreness and *pain*. If your body feels sharp pain, you may be overexerting yourself, and you could be pulling or tearing muscle. Take it easy and let your muscles recover. If you do pull a muscle, stop training immediately and begin stretching carefully and slowly. Do this several times a day for the next couple of days until the pain goes away. To prevent injuries, make sure you stretch out properly before and after your workout. If you choose to work out every other day, then on your off days, stretch out in the mornings for 10 minutes.

When cooling down from running, do not go straight to a bench and sit down. Even though you're tired, that is the worst thing you can do because it allows your muscles to tighten up. Muscles need to be slowly cooled down, rather than completely shut down. As tired as you may be, stay up and walk around slowly for at least five minutes. This will slowly cool your muscles down and prepare them to stop working.

When cooling down after swimming, use the same stretches you used before your workout. There is nothing wrong with adding to these stretches. I have included only the basic stretches and exercises. So if you learn something new from someone else, incorporate it into this workout. Just make sure you're using the proper form. The beauty of this program is that it will give you a solid foundation to build upon.

THIS PROGRAM WORKS

There's no doubt about it. I've seen it work miracles, and I know it works because it worked for me. As with anything in life, you'll get out of it what you put into it. Do not expect to achieve miraculous results working out for only 10 minutes once a week. It takes time and dedication. You purchased this book expecting a complete body workout. Well, here you go. This is the program successfully used by the finest combat forces in the world—and all you have to do is follow the instructions.

This is a time-tested, proven method for physical fitness perfection! And now it is in your hands. You can put this book on your bookshelf or throw it in your closet, and stay at your current level of fitness. Or you can tear into this book and get into the best shape of your life.

It worked for me—and it *will* work for you!

The key to your success in this program is your heart and your mind. I don't care if you are an Olympic athlete or America's #1 couch potato. If you want to become the best, remember it comes from within. I always remember the instructors asking, "Who has the fire in the gut?" If you want this so badly that you can actually feel it in your stomach, then you're on your way. You are on fire!

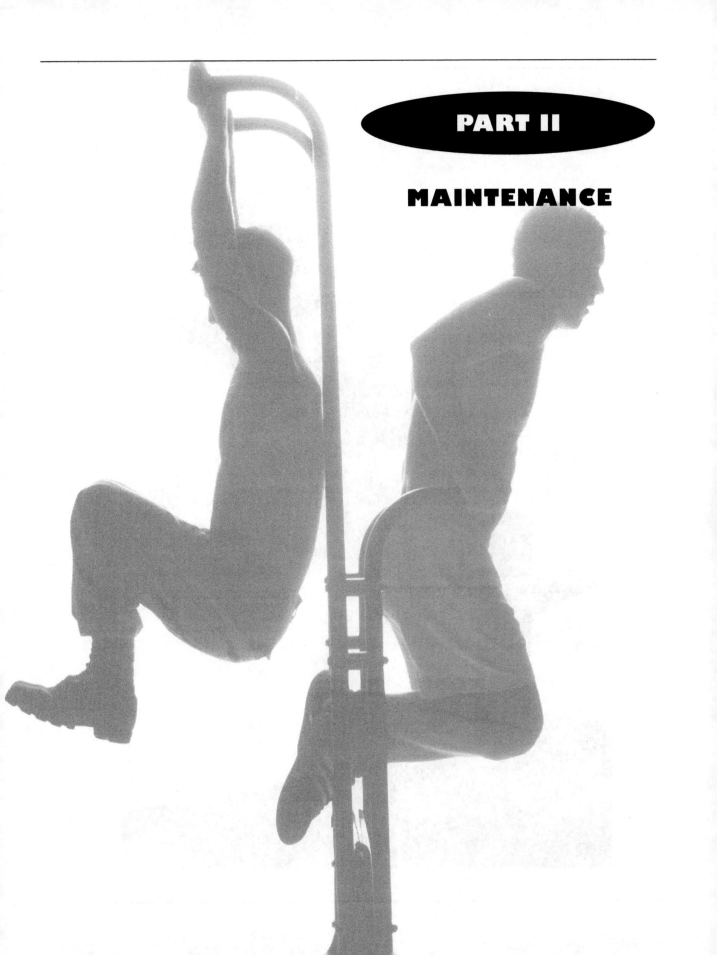

PART II

MAINTENANCE

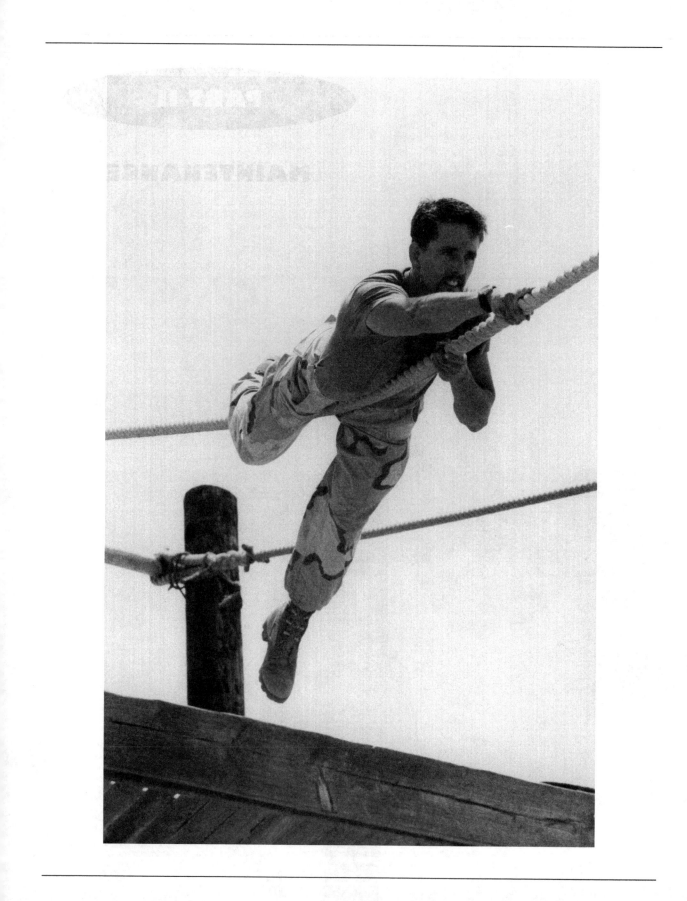

8. Diet and Nutrition

Dr. Christine DuPraw, Professor of Nutrition
Mesa College
San Diego, California

Since carbohydrates are the primary fuel for the working muscle, the diet should be rich in starches such as pasta, bread, cereals, beans, fruits, and vegetables. A good variety of foods will ensure getting enough vitamins and minerals. The USDA's Food Guide Pyramid is a useful guide to know how many servings to eat each day. Note that the foundation of the diet is carbohydrate based.

The number of servings you select should depend on your activity level and size. If you choose the maximum servings from each food group you will consume 2,800 calories. The more active you are, the more calories you will need to maintain your weight. Most people who exercise benefit from a high-carbohydrate, low-fat diet.[1] This diet would provide about 60–70 percent of the calories from carbohydrates, 15 percent from protein, and 15–25 percent from fat. Saturated animal fats like butter should be minimized and, when possible, replaced with plant oils, such as canola or peanut.

If a person does not eat a variety of foods or drops below 1,500 calories a day, he or she is at risk for malnutrition and/or vitamin deficiency. With greater physical activity, most people eat more and as long as the food is wholesome, vitamin and mineral needs will be met. In general, large doses of individual vitamins and minerals have not been shown to help an already well-nourished athlete. A person wishing to take a supplement should choose one that offers 100–200 percent of the U.S. RDA[2] of vitamins and minerals.

For individuals engaged in intense exercise, a greater intake of fruits and vegetables is advised. These foods help provide antioxidant nutrients (e.g., vitamin C and beta-carotene) which may protect the body from a potential increase of harmful free radicals. By purchasing a food composition guide or nutritional analysis software, you can figure out your calorie and nutrient intake. Remember that supplements will not take the place of a healthy diet. If you feel you need more individualized nutrition counseling, please contact SCAN[3] (sport and cardiovascular nutritionalists).

---

[1] Low-fat diet: It is recommended that people engaging in this type of diet increase their vitamin E intake to 200 I.U.
[2] United States Department of Agriculture, Recommended Daily Allowance.
[3] SCAN–Sports Nutrition Institute; telephone: (303) 779-1950.

For most people, a one-pound muscle gain per week is a reasonable goal to set. At this time it is not known how many calories are needed to make one pound of muscle tissue, nor in what form these calories should be. An estimate is that you would need to eat 400 to 500 extra calories a day to gain one pound of muscle each week. However, if you have a fast metabolism or are also participating in intense aerobic activity, you may require more calories. Be careful of caffeine and smoking—both increase metabolism.

The increase in calories should come primarily from carbohydrates, with a small increase in protein and fat. One pound of muscle is about 22 percent (100 grams) protein, 70 percent water, and 7 percent fat. Therefore, to gain one pound of muscle in a week, you would need to eat 14 grams of additional protein per day. This can easily be met by adding two cups of milk; two ounces of meat, fish, or poultry; or two ounces of cheese. Protein powders and amino acid supplements are not necessary and can be expensive. Research studies have suggested that the human body can retain only 7 to 28 grams of protein per day for muscle growth.

For athletes, another way to estimate how much protein you need is to multiply your weight in kilograms (1 pound is equal to 2.2 kilograms) by 1.5 to 1.75 grams of protein. For example, a 150-pound person would weigh 68 kilograms and should consume a maximum of 120 grams of protein each day. A three-ounce portion of meat, fish, or chicken provides about 21 grams of protein, and a cup of milk or yogurt supplies about 9 grams. Protein is easy to come by, but eating large amounts is not correlated with greater muscle development.

The remaining calories should come from whole-grain breads, cereals, pastas, and vegetables. It is very difficult for some people to gain weight unless they consume about 30 percent of their daily calories from fat. It should be emphasized that the source of this fat should come from plants rather than animals. For example, a peanut butter sandwich (avoid hydrogenated[4] peanut butter) on whole wheat bread would make a healthy, high-energy snack; a piece of broiled beef would be a less beneficial protein source. For those who get tired of always having to fix food, "liquid meals," such as Ensure and other weight-gain supplements, come in handy. A single serving can provide an additional 400 calories in a quick, easy-to-swallow formula.

TO LOSE WEIGHT

One pound of fat contains 3,500 calories. By creating a daily deficit of 500 calories, you can lose one pound of fat per week. A loss of one to two pounds per week is considered a safe weight loss. The only way to lose the fat and keep it off is to commit to

---

[4] Hydrogenation refers to the process of converting plant oil to a creamy consistency (such as margarine), which affects the texture and appearance of food products. Hydrogenated foods contain high levels of saturated fat, which raises cholesterol.

eating a low-fat diet (one in which only 20 percent or less of your caloric intake is from fat) and increasing your activity. Many people successfully lose weight by simply looking at where the fat is in their diet and substituting low- or nonfat foods. Fat provides more than twice as many calories as carbohydrates and protein. You should use caution even when eating nonfat or low-fat foods. Many nonfat baked products add extra sugar, so they are still high in calories.

Excess calories from carbohydrate, protein, or fat will cause weight gain if they're not burned in physical activity. Exercise speeds weight loss, not only by burning more calories, but by increasing metabolism due to an increase in lean body mass. The more muscle tissue developed, the more calories you will burn (even while you're relaxing). Exercise increases self-esteem, which reinforces healthy diet changes. Focus on what you can *do,* rather than what you can eat.

Here are some tips that will help you to lose weight:

- Eat breakfast.
- Drink lots of water.
- Do not eat while watching television.
- Do not eat quickly.

TO GAIN WEIGHT

A person may be underweight for a variety of reasons, e.g., medical, emotional, or hereditary. The goal in putting on weight is to gain muscle, not fat.

Here are some tips on how to gain weight successfully:

- Eat more frequently.
- Get adequate sleep and rest.
- Participate in a progressive resistance training program.

Weight training with progressively heavier weights causes the greatest stimulus to muscle development and the caloric burn is relatively small compared to more active aerobic exercise. Before starting any heavy weight-lifting program, you should have a thorough medical check-up.

The Cutting Edge
Food Guide Pyramid
A Guide to Daily Food Choices

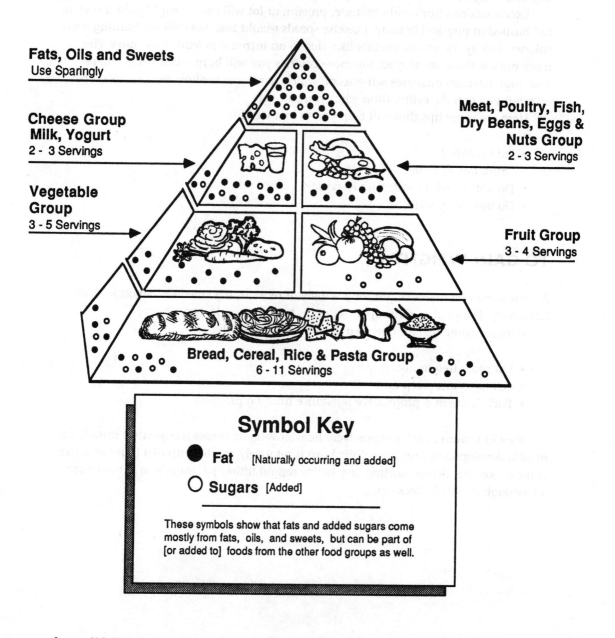

Fats, Oils and Sweets
Use Sparingly

**Cheese Group
Milk, Yogurt**
2 - 3 Servings

Vegetable Group
3 - 5 Servings

Meat, Poultry, Fish, Dry Beans, Eggs & Nuts Group
2 - 3 Servings

Fruit Group
3 - 4 Servings

Bread, Cereal, Rice & Pasta Group
6 - 11 Servings

Symbol Key

● **Fat**   [Naturally occurring and added]

○ **Sugars** [Added]

These symbols show that fats and added sugars come mostly from fats, oils, and sweets, but can be part of [or added to] foods from the other food groups as well.

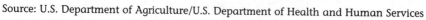

Source: U.S. Department of Agriculture/U.S. Department of Health and Human Services

The Cutting Edge
Nutrition Guide

PYRAMID FOOD GROUP	SERVING SIZE
Milk, yogurt, cheese	1 cup milk or yogurt $1^1/_2$ ounces natural cheese 2 ounces processed cheese
Meat, poultry, fish, dry beans, eggs, and nuts	2–3 ounces cooked lean meat, poultry, or fish $^1/_2$ cup cooked dry beans 1 egg 2 tablespoons peanut butter
Bread, cereal, rice, and pasta	1 slice bread 1 ounce ready-to-eat cereal $^1/_2$ cup cooked cereal, rice, or pasta
Vegetables	1 cup raw, leafy vegetables $^1/_2$ cup other vegetables, cooked or chopped raw $^3/_4$ cup vegetable juice
Fruit	1 medium apple, banana, or orange $^1/_2$ cup chopped, cooked, or canned fruit $^3/_4$ cup fruit juice
Fats, oils, sweets (Not an official food group)	None

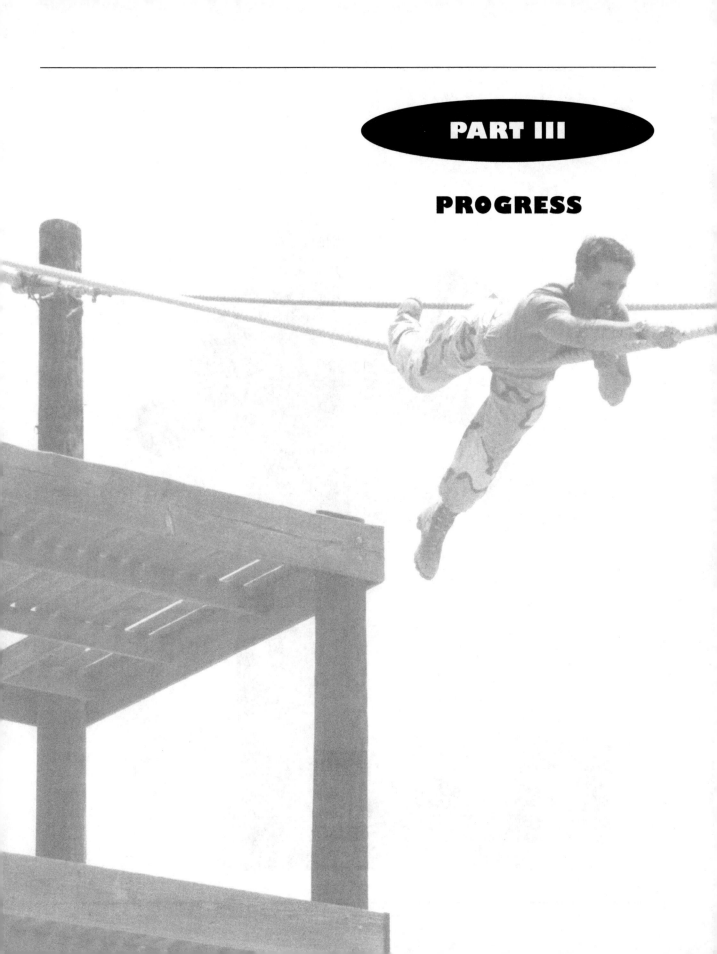

PART III

PROGRESS

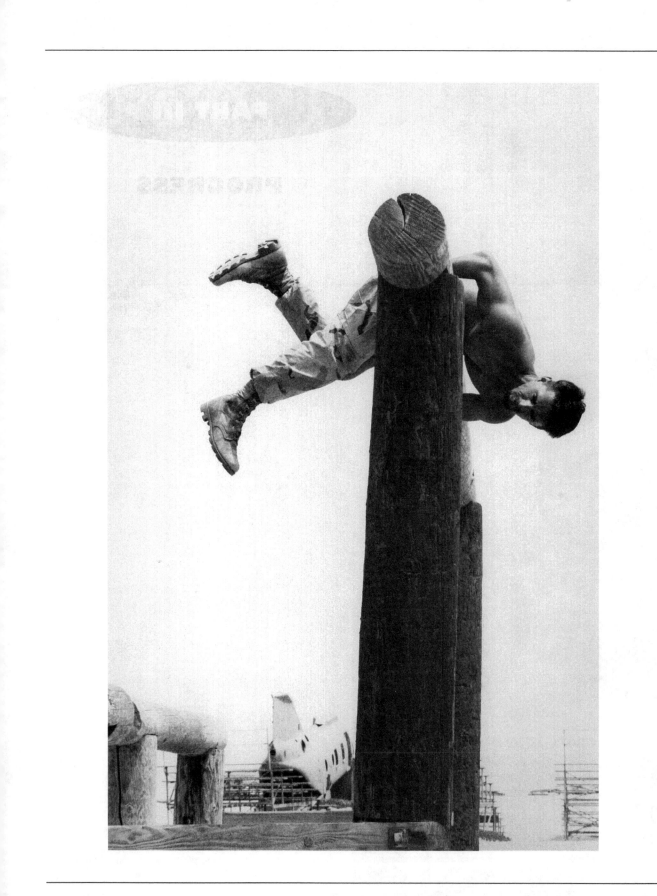

9. Progress Charts

This chapter includes three charts, which I strongly urge you to use to monitor your progress. They will keep you motivated because as you see yourself improving, you will want to continue this program with even more desire.

The first step in using these charts is to record the date you started the program, your starting weight, and the date each chart is completed. As you progress, continue to record your weight.

The second step is to do the workouts and record your starting ability for each exercise in the column labeled "Starting Ability." In a couple of months you are going to be amazed at how many repetitions you will be able to achieve.

The next step is to list your goals. As I said before, a goal not written is only a dream. Listing your goals will keep you on track for success and hold you accountable for your performance. The goal you will be shooting for on the progress charts is the number of repetitions you want to be able to perform for each individual exercise at each stage of the program. List your goal for the completion of the second week. Then list your long-term goal in the goal column on the far right. The long-term goal will be a little more difficult to predict, since it is eight weeks away.

Do not get discouraged! By the time you reach the second chart, you should be confident about reaching your long-term goal because you will be better able to predict your performance. Once you complete the second week, list your goal for the end of the fourth week. Once you complete the fourth week, list your goal for the end of the sixth week, and so on. Your short-term goals are going to be a bit more realistic than your long-term one. This is not a problem. As long as you progress steadily and improve your physical fitness, you have nothing to fear.

Other important goals for you to set are your desired weight and measurements. Before you start the program, get a measuring tape and record the starting date and your measurements. Get a friend to help you measure your waist, chest, arms, legs, and neck. Record your measurements every month thereafter, on the same day of the month. For instance, if you recorded your weight and measurements on October 8, then weigh and measure yourself again on November 8, and on the eighth day of every month thereafter. Write everything down so you can see yourself progressing on paper.

Do not get discouraged if your measurements and weight stay the same for a couple of months. Your body is adjusting to its new routine. Also, since muscle weighs more than fat, you may remain the same weight, but your waist size should go down. As your muscles grow, you are going to gain weight. At the same time, running and swimming will burn fat. So, you may remain the same weight for a few months. Again, do not get discouraged. Be happy that you are burning off excess fat—and gaining hard-earned muscle.

When you are finished with the first three charts, take the master chart and photocopy it. The blank master chart will enable you to make as many charts as you need to monitor your physical progress.

PROGRESS RECORD

Before   **After!**

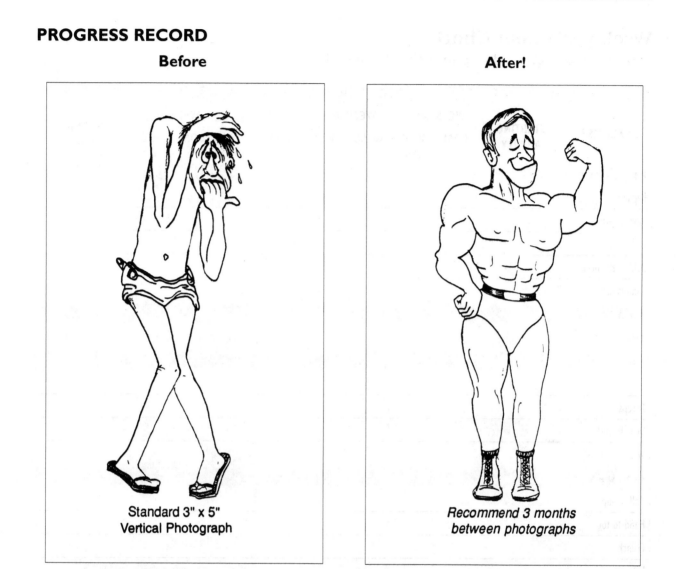

Standard 3" x 5"
Vertical Photograph

Recommend 3 months
between photographs

MEASUREMENTS

	BEFORE	3 MONTHS	6 MONTHS	9 MONTHS	AFTER!
1. Date					
2. Weight					
3. Neck					
4. Chest					
5. Biceps					
6. Triceps					
7. Waist					
8. Hips (female)					
9. Thigh					
10. Calf					

Weekly Workout Chart
Your cutting edge roadmap to a chiseled body!

EXERCISE	STARTING ABILITY	WEEK #___		WEEK #___		WEEK #___		WEEK #___		ENDING GOAL
		GOAL	ACCOM-PLISHED	GOAL	ACCOM-PLISHED	GOAL	ACCOM-PLISHED	GOAL	ACCOM-PLISHED	
PULL-UPS										
Regular										
Reverse-grip										
Close-grip										
Behind-the-neck										
Commando										
BAR DIPS										
Regular										
PUSH-UPS										
Regular										
Triceps										
Dive bomber										
Wide-angle										
SIT-UPS										
Half sit-up										
Hand-to-toe										
Crunch										
Side sit-up										
Oblique										
Flutter kick										
Leg raise										
Cutting edge										
Knee bend										
Abdominal twister										
Hanging knee-up										
Hanging leg-up										
Floor knee-up										

Weekly Workout Chart
Your cutting edge roadmap to a chiseled body!

EXERCISE	STARTING ABILITY	WEEK #___		WEEK #___		WEEK #___		WEEK #___		ENDING GOAL
		GOAL	ACCOM-PLISHED	GOAL	ACCOM-PLISHED	GOAL	ACCOM-PLISHED	GOAL	ACCOM-PLISHED	
PULL-UPS										
Regular										
Reverse-grip										
Close-grip										
Behind-the-neck										
Commando										
BAR DIPS										
Regular										
PUSH-UPS										
Regular										
Triceps										
Dive bomber										
Wide-angle										
SIT-UPS										
Half sit-up										
Hand-to-toe										
Crunch										
Side sit-up										
Oblique										
Flutter kick										
Leg raise										
Cutting edge										
Knee bend										
Abdominal twister										
Hanging knee-up										
Hanging leg-up										
Floor knee-up										

Weekly Workout Chart
Your cutting edge roadmap to a chiseled body!

EXERCISE	STARTING ABILITY	WEEK #___		WEEK #___		WEEK #___		WEEK #___		ENDING GOAL
		GOAL	ACCOM-PLISHED	GOAL	ACCOM-PLISHED	GOAL	ACCOM-PLISHED	GOAL	ACCOM-PLISHED	
PULL-UPS										
Regular										
Reverse-grip										
Close-grip										
Behind-the-neck										
Commando										
BAR DIPS										
Regular										
PUSH-UPS										
Regular										
Triceps										
Dive bomber										
Wide-angle										
SIT-UPS										
Half sit-up										
Hand-to-toe										
Crunch										
Side sit-up										
Oblique										
Flutter kick										
Leg raise										
Cutting edge										
Knee bend										
Abdominal twister										
Hanging knee-up										
Hanging leg-up										
Floor knee-up